BURNING
THE
FAT
ON
THE
FIRE

by
Lynn Montgomery
and
Margaret Thomas

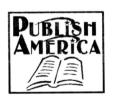

PublishAmerica
Baltimore

First printing

At the specific preference of the author, PublishAmerica allowed this work to remain exactly as the author intended, verbatim, without editorial input.

ISBN: 1-4241-9569-1
PUBLISHED BY PUBLISHAMERICA, LLLP
www.publishamerica.com
Baltimore

Printed in the United States of America

Abstain from

all appearances

of evil self-indulgence.

Scripture quotations are taken from the New Living Translation of the Holy Bible called The Book, copyright, 1996, Tyndale House Publishers, Inc. Wheaton, Illinois 60189; The Amplified Bible, copyright 1965, 1987 by the Zondervan Corporation; The Amplified New Testament copyright 1958, 1987 by The Lockman Foundation, and the King James Version.

There are many people to thank with not enough space to do it in. First and foremost we want to express our gratitude to the Lord for allowing us to write this book. He put an anointing into the wisdom He provided. Shortly after the writing of this book, Pastor David Goodwin, our Pastoral covering went home to be with the Lord. Many of the principals in the book were based on his teaching.

We want to thank our editor, Cyndy Nelson, for the long hours she spent making sure the book was readable. Her dedication transformed our manuscript into a book. We wish to thank our families for their understanding as we labored to keep our focus steady. We are grateful for the ability to work together that only the Lord could have provided.

Contents

The Press of His Fingers

The press of His fingers against my soul
Gently stripping the old man away,
Brings comfort and joy and peace to know
That Jesus is working today.
When all I surrender unto the Lord,
When all that I am I give,
When I empty myself before His throne,
That's when I begin to live.
So empty me more and then fill up my cup;
I'll be just as You would choose.
My being to You I sanctify, Lord;
My life to Your love I loose.
So, here is my life, my heart is Yours, Lord,
And all that I am is Thine.
Then He takes of my vessel and polishes bright
Till He sees Himself in the shine.

By Margaret Thomas

Foreword

"And so, dear brothers and sisters, I plead with you to give your bodies to God. Let them be a living and holy sacrifice—the kind He will accept. When you think of what He has done for you, it this too much to ask? Don't copy the behavior and customs of this world, but let God transform you into a new person by changing the way you think..." (Romans 12:1-2) New Living Translation

As you begin this forty day fast of yourself to God as a living sacrifice, burning the fat of self-indulgence on the fire of His altar, we pray for you as Paul prayed for the Ephesians, Heavenly Father, please give to all who read these words spiritual wisdom and understanding so that we will all come to know you better. Let each one be enlightened in the way they need to receive the truths held herein and be set free, amen.

Remember, this is only a devotional to help bring freedom from bondage to those who will choose to follow God's instructions from His word. It is a tool and not to be used to replace daily Bible study. It will only work if you do it because you want to and not because you have to. A living sacrifice makes conscious decisions. Anyone following a diet through the strength of his or her own will is offering dead sacrifices made under the spirit of the law. The pattern of failure is familiar to all of us who have tried it over and over again. Let's look into God's law as a mirror, see ourselves as He sees us, and choose life from Him through the Holy Spirit. This devotional is only one part of God's infinite plan to give us a future and a hope. May His blessings be upon you as you absorb these teachings and grow through them?

Preface

In the New Testament, in Matthew 11:18, John the Baptist was called demon possessed because he never drank wine and often fasted. In Matthew 11:19, Jesus was called a glutton and a drunkard because he ate and drank with sinners. We definitely need to get away from how the world sees eating and how it defines what it sees. The **world** was wrong in its observation and conclusion about both John and Jesus. The world concentrated on the outward appearance; God concentrates on the heart condition. What John did and what Jesus did were both right for them, because each one was in direct obedience to what God was telling them to do. Our success or failure depends on if we are willing to lay down our self nature and be directed by Him.

We have to stop seeing ourselves the way the world does. How would you describe yourself to someone else: short and fat; tall and heavy; or medium height, but well rounded? Think about how you picture what you look like. Begin to see yourself as God does: a beloved child; a precious son; or a daughter; a much loved, precious possession. As our focus adjusts and we begin to see God's way, we become aware of our faults, habits, and wrong choices, which are outward manifestations of inner sin. When we become willing to confess our sins, He is faithful and just to forgive us our sins and cleanse us from all unrighteousness (I John 1:9).

We have all probably dieted more than half of our lives. The results vary according to how strong we are in ourselves. How many times have we been able to follow a diet, lose weight, and reach our goal? Or we just get tired of trying and give up? Then we see it all come right back, usually with a few extra pounds added for good measure. When we set our attention on totally temporal things (a temporary fix) we just can't attain permanent weight loss. As we change our focus to eternal principles, permanent changes will be automatic.

Lynn's Testimony

I want to say right up front how I have struggled over losing weight God's way. I have probably lost a thousand pounds over my 61 years, but always through sacrifice in my flesh, and it always came back. As the Lord began to speak to my heart that I had been doing things backward, I knew I was in for some major changes. When I heard Him speak to my spirit the words to abstain from all appearances of evil self indulgence, it really hurt. He gave me the Scripture: referring to asking and receiving not, because of asking amiss, in order to consume it upon personal lusts. I immediately realized all of the times I had dieted were for the wrong reasons.

When I was younger, I remembered wanting to look sexy, wear "cool" clothes, and fit the world's image of glamour. As I got older, I wanted to feel better so I could be more active and do fun things. As the Holy Spirit began to deal with me, He let me see none of these were wrong in themselves, only in where they were in my priorities. He made me understand that putting these reasons above a desire for temperance and self-control was a form of lust. He caused me to recognize that gluttony in my life was sin and something that He hated because of the harm it brought to me. God began to say He wanted me to have my mind renewed in order for my soul to be transformed. In a nutshell, He said I was going to have to come to Him as a **living sacrifice**, asking for what I've always despised—the discipline to make the right choices over and over again, simply because they were the right choices! My motive had to become wanting to please Him and not my old fleshly self-indulgent desires. I had to realize when I came to Him this way; He would always give me His perfect answer. I had to come to an understanding that I didn't have to do this, but I would be glad if I did. I would come to a place where I would be grateful for the disciplining, and I wouldn't want to go back to my old ways. Those ways seemed right to me, but the end was death. Now I realized that the death I had to experience was the death to self, which makes me alive to God. I had to relinquish this part of my life into His control and make Jesus Lord of my weight loss, too.

The Lord showed me the tabernacle He called the Israelites to build in the wilderness. He reminded me that we are now the temple (tabernacle) of the Holy Spirit, and He lives in us. I saw the two rooms of the tabernacle, the Holy Place and the most Holy Place. I read in the Old Testament how the Holy Place was used for daily sacrifice, cleansing, repentance, and fellowship. I saw how the most Holy Place could only be accessed by the high priest and then only once a year. He let me see how the curtain between the two rooms had been torn in half through Jesus' blood sacrifice on the cross. We were given bold access to the most Holy Place from that time on. I began to realize that I was continuing to live only in the Holy Place. I was going over and over again into a sacrificial mode of giving things to Him when He was saying, "I desire obedience and not sacrifice." He showed me it is only in His presence that we experience power, change, intimacy, and anointing. This anointing is what destroys every yoke of bondage.

I was beginning to see the difference in what I had been doing through dieting and what God was calling me to do now in obedience. I could no longer work on outward actions, but I had to allow Him to begin to change inner motives. I saw how in the daily sacrifices of animals in that old tabernacle, the special fat that surrounded the innermost parts of the animals were always burned on the altar. God reminded me that He is an all-consuming fire. Just as the fire in that tabernacle never went out, neither does the fire of the Holy Spirit within our lives. I, as a living sacrifice, needed to die to myself and become alive to Him. This happens to us as we embrace the perfect sacrifice of Jesus Christ on the Cross and are cleansed by His blood. I had to allow the fire of God to burn away the fatness of my self-indulgence on a daily basis. I realized that I must do this for the rest of my life (not just until I reached my goal weight) if I wanted to live a victorious life. This would be the end of my self-directed life and the beginning of an eternal God-directed life of discipline. I knew this was where my victory began. My expectation became not just looking good and feeling better, but the absolute knowing that I would have a new relationship with Him. I would reap the benefit of a greater intimacy along with having consistency and stability worked into my character. Losing weight would be the outward result of these inner changes.

I saw outward fatness switching to inward fatness. My body was losing fat and my spirit was gaining it. This picture became so clear: I saw my soul getting fatter and fatter until the yoke of bondage no longer fit and it broke off (Isaiah 27:10). In Deuteronomy 32:15, God talks about fat, unruly people. In Isaiah 10:27 He talks about the anointed fatness that causes our spirit to enlarge until the yoke of bondage around our souls does not fit any more. It actually prevents the yoke from ever fitting again if we continue in obedience. Paul said in 2 Corinthians 12:9, "...Therefore, I will all the more gladly glory in my weakness and infirmities, that the strength and power of Christ (the Messiah) may rest, (yes, may pitch a tent [tabernacle] over and dwell) upon me." (Amplified)

I needed to remind myself that in the wilderness wandering the Israelites murmured and complained continually. They announced their doubt and unbelief to God and hated His discipline. They were kept from entering into their promised land because of this. Our old nature that hates the disciplining of the Lord will rise up wanting to murmur and complain, too. Mind did! (And still does if I give it half a chance.) When this happens, arm yourself with praise. I might suggest you find some music that helps you get into a praise mode. I have found Ric Gorden, born again Jewish singer and songwriter, to provide this in a wonderful way. To keep the murmuring and complaining away, it helps to start with praising God.

Get sick with me of revisiting the same old defeats! Let discipline become a beautiful word in your vocabulary. See it as a fruit of the Spirit and one that you want to remain! Let's believe that what is impossible with man is possible with God (Matthew 19:26). We can see this as a never-ending and new adventure. We will never arrive as long as we are here in this world, but we can certainly make our journey to the Promised Land more enjoyable.

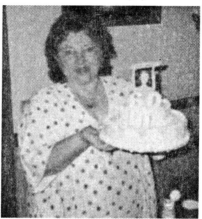

Before

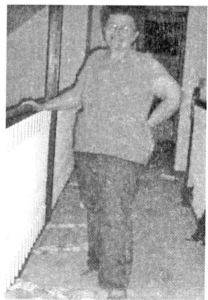

After

—Day 1—
Be Filled with the Spirit

Daily Opening Prayer

Heavenly Father, I come to you in the name of my Lord, Jesus Christ to present myself as a living sacrifice, which is my reasonable service. Cleanse me today from the sin of willfulness and fill me with your holiness. Today, I choose to burn the fat on the fire. Accept this offering and enable me to live a self-controlled life by the power of the Holy Spirit who lives in me. I refuse to despise and resist the disciplining of the Lord, which demonstrates His great love for me. We ask this in Jesus' name, amen.

As we have prayed and written these pages, we have become very aware of the necessity to be filled daily with the Holy Spirit of God. It seems only fair that we give the first day to Him. After all, He is the one who makes it all happen! Actually, His presence is absolutely necessary in each devotional teaching: to enlighten, empower and encourage us to go on. The fulfillment of every promise given to us in both the Old and New Testaments is made possible by the indwelling presence of the Holy Spirit.

We are told that before the foundations of the world, God's plan was complete for our lives. His intention, from the beginning, was to fellowship with His creation. When we believe in Jesus, God's perfect sacrifice, God is able to forgive and cleanse us from all sin. The Holy Spirit baptizes us into Jesus. Every believer is brought alive from the death of sin and has God's own Spirit dwelling in him through this operation of God. (Read Colossians 2:6-23.) In verse 6 we are reminded that in the same way we received Christ Jesus, we are to continue in Him. Remember, it is all by faith. We hear God's Word, we believe it and do it, and the Holy Spirit makes it happen. We are relieved of the pressure of trying to make it happen ourselves.

17

Through salvation, our spirit is born again into the life flow of God. We are told in 1 Thessalonians 5:23 that we are a spirit, we have a soul and we live in a body. By allowing Jesus to baptize us in the Holy Spirit, the power of the Godhead is made available to our souls. It is what the soul decides that is acted out in the body. It is absolutely necessary to bring the spirit and the soul into agreement. This is what we will do during this 40-day time of change.

Let's picture an old house that gets a complete renovation. It is made new in every area. All of the inner wiring has to be brought up to code. This is exactly what happens to us when we're born again. "Therefore if any man be in Christ, he is a new creature: old things are passed away; behold, all things are become new." (2 Corinthians 5:17) King James Version

Now picture this house with all this power run into it and made available, but the owner continues to use candles and a fireplace. The new refrigerator, air conditioning, lighting, television, or computers are useless because no one has released the power. It is the same in our lives. Just as the homeowner has to have an electrician do this, we have to have Jesus to release the indwelling power of God out of our spirits and into our souls. We are promised that as we walk in the spirit we will not fulfill the lusts of our flesh (Galatians 5:16). The fulfillment of our fleshly lusts is evident every time we look in a mirror.

If you have never received Jesus as your Savior, now is the perfect time to accept Him. Romans 10:9-10 tells us that if you will confess with your mouth Jesus as your Lord and believe in your heart that God raised Him from the dead, you will be saved. If you have never asked Jesus to release the power of God from your spirit into your soul, you can do this now, too. Just ask Him to baptize you in the Holy Spirit (Matthew 3:11).

During the next forty days, remember God has made available to you everything you need to be changed. These changes will go on through the rest of your life and into eternity. As you remain submitted and surrendered, you will see your life change in remarkable ways. You will lose weight and keep it off. The Holy

Spirit is the One given to us to help us work out salvation in every area of our lives. He shows us from the Word what is available to us in Jesus Christ. He works in us both to desire God's best and then to make us able to receive it.

Prayer

Heavenly Father, I thank you for your way of salvation through Jesus Christ. Thank you, Jesus, for being obedient. Thank you for making available to me through your death, burial and resurrection, the indwelling presence of the Holy Spirit. Forgive me for not taking full advantage of all you have provided. Today, I choose to surrender to you as both Savior and Lord. I praise You and thank You that You, Holy Spirit, are working in me to guide me and make me able. I know as I remain obedient, I will see my life transformed and my body loses weight. We ask this in Jesus' name, amen.

—Day 2—
You Are a New Creature

Daily Opening Prayer

Heavenly Father, I come to you in the name of my Lord, Jesus Christ to present myself as a living sacrifice, which is my reasonable service. Cleanse me today from the sin of willfulness and fill me with your holiness. Today, I choose to burn the fat on the fire. Accept this offering and enable me to live a self-controlled life by the power of the Holy Spirit who lives in me. I refuse to despise and resist the disciplining of the Lord, which demonstrates His great love for me. We ask this in Jesus' name, amen.

In today's society the cares of this world seem to come at us from every direction at once. They beat us up, put us down, and try to bury us with no hope for something better. Because we have been conditioned by these outward attacks it is hard to see beyond them to the very heart of our problem. We overeat, feel guilty, look awful, and continually reaffirm that this is the way it's always going to be. Thank God that He has sent us a way out.

The Bible tells us that Jesus is the Way—the Truth—and—the Life. He shows us the way, He tells us the truth, and He gives us the life. In 2 Corinthians 5:17 we are told that when we become Christians we become new persons. We are not the same anymore. The old life is gone and a new life has begun. No one is going to be successful as a new creation unless they realize they must start over from the point of their new birth and learn everything God's way. Even Jesus told His disciples that unless they became as little children they would never get into the Kingdom of Heaven (Matthew 18:3-4).

If this is the new way we have to learn, how do we do it? If we are new persons, how do we find the path of this new walk? The Bible tells us in Romans 8:14 that all who are led by the Spirit of God are the children of God. So, it is not by observing outward rules and regulations, but by an inward yielding of our hearts to God that we are able to begin this new life. We read, "And now, just as you accepted Christ Jesus as your Lord, you must continue to live in obedience to him. Let your roots grow down into him and draw up nourishment from him, so you will grow in faith, strong and vigorous in the truth you were taught. Let your lives overflow with thanksgiving for all he has done." (Colossians 2:6-7) New Living Translation

God's plan for us begins at rebirth in Jesus by God's own Spirit coming to live inside of us. Now, we are able to choose to follow God because with the born-again experience, we are dead to our sins. (Read Romans 6:17). It is important to understand that we can also make choices in our lives that render this born again nature of no effect. Remember, there is only no condemnation for those who are in Christ Jesus who walk after the Spirit and not after the flesh (Romans 8:1).

The way we grow up into successful, mature believers is by denying our flesh and following God's Spirit. He will teach us from God's Word how to live. We will then please God and ourselves. We will see ourselves as He sees us and become the reflection of His love we were always intended to be.

We can also have a new start in our weight loss attempts, not by following rigid rules, but by God's own Spirit teaching us moderation.

Prayer

Heavenly Father, I thank you that you have made me a new person in Christ Jesus and given me a brand new start. Forgive me when I forget this and return to my old habits. Holy Spirit, help me to make the right choices. Today, I will be obedient to the word, which will nourish my spirit and cause me to grow in Christ. My body will lose weight as a result of my inward obedience. I praise you and thank you for this victory. We ask this in Jesus' name, amen.

—Day 3—
The Destructive Force of Overeating

Daily Opening Prayer

Heavenly Father, I come to you in the name of my Lord, Jesus Christ to present myself as a living sacrifice, which is my reasonable service. Cleanse me today from the sin of willfulness and fill me with your holiness. Today, I choose to burn the fat on the fire. Accept this offering and enable me to live a self-controlled life by the power of the Holy Spirit who lives in me. I refuse to despise and resist the disciplining of the Lord, which demonstrates His great love for me. We ask this in Jesus' name, amen.

How often do we stop and really look at the devastation overeating has brought on our lives? Diseases of every kind find an open door into our bodies. It is the same door that we use to keep stuffing ourselves. The damages are twofold. Our bodies suffer, but so do our souls. We live beaten down, miserable, and defeated lives because we keep making choices that are destroying us.

We read, "It seems to be a fact of life that when I want to do what is right, I inevitably do what is wrong."(Romans 7:21) New Living Translation God knows how weak we are and even spells it out for us here in Romans. He is not only aware of our struggle, but His compassion and love desires to see us set free. At this point we must make a conscious decision to go on living in our misery or ask God to help us gain our freedom. The Bible tells in 1 Corinthians 10:13 that the tests that we face in our lives aren't any different from what others go through. It tells us that God is faithful. He will keep the tests from becoming so strong that we can't stand up against them. In the midst of every test, the temptation to sin will come. The test itself is the overall circumstance. When we start fighting against the circumstances, we are doing it in the flesh. We just want the problem to go away. God allows these into our lives because He knows they are the tools which will bring about permanent change if we submit ourselves to this discipline. It is through resisting the temptation to get out of the test itself that we find our way to escape. The test cannot destroy us, but giving into the temptation to get out of it can.

What we don't like in the midst of the test are the two things it points out: how weak our faith is and how strong our flesh is. At this point, if we will yield to the Lord and resist the temptation to sin by running from the test, God will cause our faith to grow stronger and our flesh to die. Even though the circumstances are still there, we are carried on through to the end by our faith in Him.

If we really want to turn away from the destructive force of overeating, we have to make a conscious choice to put down the flesh and actually ask for a time of testing. A fast is when you purposely offer yourself as a living sacrifice. You make a decision that you are deliberately going to deny your fleshly appetites for food and submit yourself to God until you know the destructive force of overeating has been broken over your life.

In 1 Peter 4:1-2 we are told: "So then, since Christ suffered physical pain, you must arm yourselves with the same attitude He had, and be ready to suffer, too. For if you are willing to suffer for Christ, you have decided to stop sinning. And you won't spend the rest of your life chasing after evil desires, but you will be anxious to do the will of God." (New Living Translation) We realize as our flesh begins to die we start to rejoice in the sense of freedom from sin. It has been made possible by enduring the process. The focus must be on the Lord and not on dieting. If we have a fleshly reason for losing weight, we always end up in failure. Sooner or later, our appetites take over; we end up still in bondage, gaining it all back. If, through the Spirit, we put to death the negative actions of our bodies we will be set free forever.

Prayer
Heavenly Father, I thank you for showing me how to break the power of the destructive force that overeating has on my life. Forgive

me for choosing to remain in this bondage. Forgive me for choosing to live in misery, rather than accept your way out. Today, I will deny my fleshly appetites, present myself to you as a living sacrifice and be set free. I will resist the temptation to get out of this discipline. I praise you and thank you that through this process you will change me from the inside out. We ask this in Jesus' name, amen.

—Day 4—
Burning the Fat on the Fire

Daily Opening Prayer

Heavenly Father, I come to you in the name of my Lord, Jesus Christ to present myself as a living sacrifice, which is my reasonable service. Cleanse me today from the sin of willfulness and fill me with your holiness. Today, I choose to burn the fat on the fire. Accept this offering and enable me to live a self-controlled life by the power of the Holy Spirit who lives in me. I refuse to despise and resist the disciplining of the Lord, which demonstrates His great love for me. We ask this in Jesus' name, amen.

God tells us we are the temple of the Holy Spirit (2 Corinthians 6:16). The temple was where offerings were brought and burned on the fire. The type of offering was made according to the need of the person or congregation. No matter what type of animal offering it was, the fat from around the kidneys, liver, and any of the innermost organs was always burned on the fire. The significance here reveals God's desire for the most intimate parts of our lives to be totally given over to Him.

Offerings were public and private, but all offerings of animal sacrifices required the shedding of blood. The Bible tells us that without the shedding of blood there is no remission of sin. Our personal sins have been washed away, because Jesus, as the perfect sacrifice, presented His own blood at the mercy seat in Heaven. This was done once, for all who would believe and receive it. This sacrifice provided our entrance into the most Holy Place.

We can now daily meet God within this temple in which we live; we no longer have to offer blood. Jesus did that. Daily, we offer to God peace offerings. These always demanded that the fat be burned on the fire. God is an all-consuming fire in our lives, and it pleases

Him greatly as we freely choose to do this. We are set free from any need to sacrifice for sin, though we must daily confess our sins so His blood can cleanse us from all unrighteousness.

The fat that was burned by the priests was considered the choicest, finest, richest part of an animal sacrifice. When we daily, as priests ourselves now, give God the gift of ourselves as a living sacrifice, He begins to burn the fat from our hearts, which has dulled our relationship with Him. Each time the Old Testament priests burned the fat on the fire, they were putting God first. As we put God first in our daily lives and choose to obey Him in His commands, He not only burns away the inner fat of self-indulgence, but also the outward fat on our bodies. We call this process dieting. God will produce an inward, permanent change which will result in an outward weight loss from our bodies.

Prayer

Heavenly Father, I thank you for explaining your word so I can understand it and do it. Forgive me for being lazy and self-indulgent. Today, I choose to offer myself to you as a living sacrifice. Please burn the fat on the fire from my inner man and my outer man. I praise you that as I continue being obedient to your word, I will see my life become disciplined and my body will lose weight. We ask this in Jesus' name, amen.

—Day 5—

Judgment Begins First at the House of God (Whose House We Are)

Daily Opening Prayer

Heavenly Father, I come to you in the name of my Lord, Jesus Christ to present myself as a living sacrifice, which is my reasonable service. Cleanse me today from the sin of willfulness and fill me with your holiness. Today, I choose to burn the fat on the fire. Accept this offering and enable me to live a self-controlled life by the power of the Holy Spirit who lives in me. I refuse to despise and resist the disciplining of the Lord, which demonstrates His great love for me. We ask this in Jesus' name, amen.

The Bible tells us that the time for judgment has come and it must start with God's people (1 Peter 4:17). None of us, in the natural sense, likes to have someone judge us. It usually makes us angry and resentful. It leaves us with a stubborn sense of "who do they think they are?" We then go out and do exactly what we were told was the wrong thing to do. And who ends up the loser? Not the person offering the judgment. We lose the battle, eat too much of the wrong things, and gain more weight.

Sometimes judgment comes from a mean-spirited person who's just trying to hurt us. This would not be from God, but He can use it for good if we choose to let Him. Other times, God uses someone whose heart is full of love to offer a judgment that is filled with truth. In John 8:32 Jesus told His disciples that they would know the truth and the truth would set them free. Proverbs 16:6 says that through mercy and truth, iniquity or sin is purged.

Judgment starts first of all as a word of correction. This is why it has to begin first at the House of God. Only God's own people recognize His voice. However, sometimes we are stubborn and refuse to listen. We want the blessing to be on our way of doing things without having to change and do things God's way. Because

He loves us so much, God allows warning signs to caution us in our self-indulgence. We get short of breath, we become lethargic, we have pain in our knees and hips from carrying too much weight, and we find ourselves sitting around watching others do the things we used to enjoy. Again, we have the choice. Do we heed these warnings or do we continue on in our own ways? When we resist God's judgment we compound our problem by adding disobedience and rebellion to it.

God told King Saul that rebellion was as bad as the sin of witchcraft and stubbornness was as bad as worshiping idols (1 Samuel 15:23). Whenever God brings correction, it is because He desires to see us set free from bondages in our lives. We must see that if we are truly God's children He has the right and responsibility to bring this correction. (Read Hebrews 12:6-11).

We must also see that any correction God brings into our life is for our benefit and motivated by His great love for us. God always works to set His own people free first. We, then, in turn can be used to reach out in love to help others. What better way for people to see a change in our lives than when they see us lose weight permanently? God can use this as an opportunity for us to share our testimony and help someone else who is struggling through where we have just come.

In 2 Corinthians 1:3-4 the Bible tells us to praise God because He is the source of every mercy and the one who comforts us in all of our troubles. When we have received God's judgment in our lives and have been corrected by it, we are made able to reach out to others with His compassion and authority.

Prayer

Heavenly Father, I thank you for your judgment, as I submit myself to you that begin first in my life. You are correcting me because I belong to you. Forgive me when I am stubborn and rebellious and resist your correction. Help me to quit resisting and surrender completely. Today, I will welcome your guidance in my life. I praise you because your judgment always brings deliverance. I am being changed into your image both inside and out. We ask this in Jesus' name, amen.

—Day 6—
Arm Yourself with the Mind of Christ

Daily Opening Prayer

Heavenly Father, I come to you in the name of my Lord, Jesus Christ to present myself as a living sacrifice, which is my reasonable service. Cleanse me today from the sin of willfulness and fill me with your holiness. Today, I choose to burn the fat on the fire. Accept this offering and enable me to live a self-controlled life by the power of the Holy Spirit who lives in me. I refuse to despise and resist the disciplining of the Lord, which demonstrates His great love for me. We ask this in Jesus' name, amen.

How many times do we think, *this is just too much, nobody can stand this kind of tribulation. We're supposed to be God's children. I would never treat my kids this way!* First and foremost we need to establish the fact that God is love. The problem lies in our total misconception of what this really means. We judge God's love to be conditional, like ours. The truth is we have tried to bring God down to our level of existence. It will never happen. Where we are limited to our immediate circumstances for information, God sees timelessly into the past, present and future all at the same time. He always has our best in mind, but sometimes because of our own choices, we suffer needlessly.

God, in His wisdom, decided to leave tribulation in this world. He could have dealt with it the same way He dealt with sin, but He chose to allow it in our lives because He knew He could use it to accomplish His purposes. In John 16:33 we are told that in this world we would have tribulation, but we are to be cheerful about it. We are told that Jesus overcame the world. We are told that He learned obedience through the things that He suffered. How can we learn the same obedience in any way except the one that was used on Him?

29

Let's think of tribulation as God's gymnasium. In the natural when we go to the gym to exercise, we experience a certain amount of discomfort. No Pain—No Gain. As we submit to the training, two things happen. First, our muscles are exercised and gain strength. Second, if we don't give up and quit, we lose body fat.

It is the same in God's Gym. When we submit to His discipline in the midst of tribulation, two things happen also. First, our faith is tried (exercised) and made stronger. Secondly, as our flesh is tempted and we resist the temptation, our flesh begins to die. Initially, what we hate about both kinds of workouts is that we become aware of how weak we are. Most of the time we avoid the very things that can make us strong and accomplish our hearts' desire to be changed into the image of Christ in our inner man and lose weight from our outward man.

In 1 Peter 4:1-3 we read, "So then, since Christ suffered physical pain, you must arm yourselves with the same attitude He had, and be ready to suffer, too. For if you are willing to suffer for Christ, you have decided to stop sinning. And you won't spend the rest of your life chasing after evil desires, but you will be anxious to do the will of God." (New Living Translation) If we really want to see God's answers in our desire to lose weight, we must stop avoiding the discomfort of tribulation. In fact, we must willingly choose it as part of our lifestyle. If we do this we will gain strength and lose flesh, both inwardly and outwardly, through the operation of God.

Prayer

Heavenly Father, I want to thank you for instructing me that not to fear tribulations. Forgive me when I try to avoid rather than embrace what you are allowing in my life to make me strong. Today, I willingly exercise my faith and deny my flesh. I praise you that as I do this, you will be at work in me to change me inside and out. We ask this in Jesus' name, amen.

—Day 7—
Getting into God's Flow

Daily Opening Prayer

Heavenly Father, I come to you in the name of my Lord, Jesus Christ to present myself as a living sacrifice, which is my reasonable service. Cleanse me today from the sin of willfulness and fill me with your holiness. Today, I choose to burn the fat on the fire. Accept this offering and enable me to live a self-controlled life by the power of the Holy Spirit who lives in me. I refuse to despise and resist the disciplining of the Lord, which demonstrates His great love for me. I ask this in Jesus' name, amen.

Recently, my husband and I had the opportunity to fly to Oregon from our home in Orlando, Florida. Getting between gates in a timely manner has always been a challenge, but with each passing year, it seems to become more of one. We needed to go from one concourse to another and it was a long way! We were so thankful for the "moving sidewalks." What a relief to just step on and be taken where we needed to go without having to struggle to get there. It reminded us of how God wants us to get into the flow of His "moving sidewalk."

After greeting the believers, Paul interjects a wonderful promise in Philippians chapter one. He tells them of his complete confidence that the work God has begun in them, God will see through to its finish. This promise includes all of us today. God is not going to leave us stuck with no way to reach our destination. Let us remember that each new day brings opportunity for new commitment. He won't force us into His flow, but He will help us in each temptation to run away, so that we have His way to escape. Our part is to set our will to enter into His flow. Once we have done this He makes His power available to carry us along.

We are told we can do all things through Christ who gives us the strength (Philippians 4:13). Our desire to stay in God's flow stops when our flesh rebels against the discipline He is using to change us. We begin with a desire to present ourselves to the Lord as a living sacrifice. We get excited when we see a weight loss, because of this inner commitment beginning to work. As time passes, weight loss slows down because there is a natural, bodily resistance to losing weight too quickly. What we fail to remember is it took several years to gain the extra pounds we are carrying. We want to lose it all in a few months time with the least amount of effort. Rather than murmuring and complaining because the outward change has slowed, let us use this time as an opportunity to recommit ourselves to the reason we started, presenting ourselves to God as that living sacrifice. Even here, we have God's help. In Philippians 2:13 Paul reminds us that God is working in us, giving us the desire to obey Him and the power to do what pleases Him. What a wonderful Father we have! He has left nothing out. This is why we have confidence that as we commit ourselves into His flow He will carry us through to His perfect end. When we exercise our faith, we begin to see ourselves as He see us, changed into the image of His Son. As we inwardly delight ourselves in Him, He will give us the desire of our hearts. When we commit our way unto the Lord, trusting in Him, He will bring it to pass (Psalm 37:4-5).

Prayer

Heavenly Father, I thank you for providing a flow of power through Jesus Christ that begin and finish your work in me. Forgive me when I step out of this flow and complain that it's too hard. Today, I will delight myself in you. I will commit my way to you. As I do this, you will work in my heart and life to change my inner man and my outward appearance. Weight loss will happen as a direct result of my obedience. How I praise and thank you for your faithfulness. I ask this in Jesus' name, amen.

—Day 8—
He Gives Fresh Manna Daily

Daily Opening Prayer

Heavenly Father, I come to you in the name of my Lord, Jesus Christ to present myself as a living sacrifice, which is my reasonable service. Cleanse me today from the sin of willfulness and fill me with your holiness. Today, I choose to burn the fat on the fire. Accept this offering and enable me to live a self-controlled life by the power of the Holy Spirit who lives in me. I refuse to despise and resist the disciplining of the Lord, which demonstrates His great love for me. I ask this in Jesus' name, amen.

In the Old Testament we read how God provided manna daily for the physical needs of the Israelites. However, the minds of the people were so intent on what was being provided that they forgot to bless and rejoice in their Providence. In Jesus' day, people were still intent on gratifying their immediate needs. He had to address the problem in Matthew 6:25-34. He told the people not to worry about their everyday life—what they were going to eat, what they were going to drink, or what they would wear. He reminded them of their heavenly Father who knew they needed these things and wanted to provide them.

People are still pretty much the same today. How many times is our first waking thought about food? The minute awareness hits, our minds say to us, *here's a new day, and what will we eat in it?* The Bible tells us how we should start each day, "This is the day the Lord has made, we will rejoice and be glad in it." (Psalms 118:24) New Living Translation All through the ages, people have been afraid to trust God to provide what they needed. From the very beginning, God has done nothing but provide. God gives us our food, as we need it; He opens His hand and satisfies the hunger and thirst of every living thing (Psalms 145:15-16).

The problem seems to rest with the fact that there are two kinds of hunger at work within us: physical and spiritual. We need to recognize that the real manna we need is the bread that came down from Heaven, Jesus Himself. He alone will satisfy the inner hunger we all feel.

In America we're not really afraid we won't get enough to eat; we're just afraid we won't get what we really want. Our old natures have been so indulged that they are very powerful and demand to keep on being fed in the same manner they have been used to. If we will first feed our inner man each day by feasting on God's Word and drinking in His presence, it will become easier to make wise choices as to what we will eat in the natural. Remember, man can't live by bread alone, but by every word that comes forth from the mouth of God (Deuteronomy 8:3; Matthew 4:4).

Prayer

Heavenly Father, thank you that I can trust you to provide all that I have need of today. I know your provision is always perfect. Forgive me when I forget to eat of your word and put all of my focus on filling my stomach. Today, I will fill my soul first. I praise you that you are sufficient for all of my daily needs. I ask this in Jesus' name, amen.

—Day 9—

Do Not Be Discouraged—Is Anything Too Hard for the Lord?

Daily Opening Prayer

Heavenly Father, I come to you in the name of my Lord, Jesus Christ to present myself as a living sacrifice, which is my reasonable service. Cleanse me today from the sin of willfulness and fill me with your holiness. Today, I choose to burn the fat on the fire. Accept this offering and enable me to live a self-controlled life by the power of the Holy Spirit who lives in me. I refuse to despise and resist the disciplining of the Lord, which demonstrates His great love for me. I ask this in Jesus' name, amen.

How often has repeated failure in dieting made you feel so helpless, hopeless and totally unworthy that you can't even begin to picture success? Let us consider the story of father Abraham who by faith followed God and was blessed abundantly. In the midst of all of these innumerable blessings, one day he cried out to God, "What good are all these blessings when I have no child?" God then promised to fulfill the desire of Abraham's heart. You know the rest of the story. At 100 years of age, Abraham finally received the child of the promise.

Have we not in like manner sat and listened to some preacher tell us how God wants to satisfy the desire of our hearts only to immediately be reminded that we've prayed over and over again to lose weight, but it just doesn't happen? Like Abraham and Sarah, nothing we try seems to help. They even got the bright idea to use a surrogate mother. They brought their servant girl, Hagar, to Abraham and a son was born. However, there was no peace, contentment, or enjoyment in him. Then God came to Abraham again and told him he would indeed have a son through his wife Sarah. When Sarah heard this she laughed. They both had settled for the best they could do, but God wanted to give them His best. God's word to them was: "Is anything too hard for the Lord?" (Genesis 18:14). New Living Translation

In the area of weight control, we are settling for the best we can do without realizing that God has something better. Are we living without peace, contentment, and joy because we haven't seen His whole answer? Abraham and Sarah had become so discouraged because so much time had passed. They thought the son Abraham had conceived with Hagar was the only one that God was offering. Then God came to them in their old age and said, "I'm going to give you and Sarah a son." Is it any wonder they had a hard time believing it?

How many of us are in our forties, fifties, sixties, or even older and have become so discouraged with dieting that just living where we are is better than yo-yoing back and forth in our weight? Have we become so tired of it all we say, "Why even try?" Surprisingly, this is exactly where God wants us to be! Now, His strength can be made perfect in our weakness. The things that are impossible for us are possible with God.

He takes delight in remembering and answering the deepest cry of our hearts. As we surrender, His answer becomes possible. Let's stop laughing it off, like Sarah did, and submit ourselves to God's greatness. He will meet us where we are and bring us to where we desire to be. As He changes us inside, outward weight loss will happen as surely as Abraham and Sarah received the child of promise. Not only will we have the outward answer, we will have a deeper relationship with our God.

Prayer

Heavenly Father, I thank you that nothing is impossible with you. Forgive me that I have been living satisfied with what I can do. Today, I will quit laughing it off, and allow you, Holy Spirit, to help me believe I can lose weight. I praise you that what's important to me is important to you and you want me to have the full benefit of your promises. I thank you, in Jesus' name, amen.

—Day 10—
Come as a Child

Daily Opening Prayer

Heavenly Father, I come to you in the name of my Lord, Jesus Christ to present myself as a living sacrifice, which is my reasonable service. Cleanse me today from the sin of willfulness and fill me with your holiness. Today, I choose to burn the fat on the fire. Accept this offering and enable me to live a self-controlled life by the power of the Holy Spirit who lives in me. I refuse to despise and resist the disciplining of the Lord, which demonstrates His great love for me. We ask this in Jesus' name, amen.

How many of us learned most of our ingrained habits as children? This includes the good and the bad ones. The Bible says, "Train up a child in the way he should go and when he is grown, he will not depart from it." One of the most endearing traits a child demonstrates is their trust and acceptance. How often have our hearts melted when sons or daughters hold up their little arms to be held "just because." On the other hand, how grievous is it when that closeness is broken by disobedience?

In Matthew 18:2, Jesus, while his disciples were arguing over who was greatest, calls a little child into their midst. He gives them a warning that unless they would become as this little child, they would never get into the Kingdom of Heaven. This willingness to humble ourselves doesn't stop with being born again. It affects every part of our lives.

God tells us in Isaiah 55 that His thoughts are not our thoughts and His ways are not our ways. The scripture says in Proverbs 14:12 that there is a way that seems right to a man, but the end of this way leads to death. Have you found that, because of the conditioning you received as a child, your eating habits are leading you toward destruction? Do you still hear, "Clean your plate, there are children starving all over the world"? Were you rewarded with food for being good? Were you encouraged to "eat, it's good for you"? God wants to break the power of these habits over our lives. He has a new and better way. To learn this new way, we must come to Him as little children. We must be willing to trust Him and be teachable. As He instructs us in this new way of life, He changes us in our inner man and we lose weight as an outward result of this change.

Prayer

Heavenly Father, thank you for the way that you have for me that lead to life and health. Forgive me when I think my ways are better than yours. I confess that my ways are how I've gotten so out of control in my appetites. Today, I will come to you, trusting you as a child. I will be obedient to your instruction. I am willing to be teachable. I praise you that as your new way changes me inwardly, I will see my body lose weight as a consequence of this obedience. I ask this in Jesus' name, amen.

—Day 11—
What Happened at the Altar Must Be Implemented in Our Lives

Daily Opening Prayer

Heavenly Father, I come to you in the name of my Lord, Jesus Christ to present myself as a living sacrifice, which is my reasonable service. Cleanse me today from the sin of willfulness and fill me with your holiness. Today, I choose to burn the fat on the fire. Accept this offering and enable me to live a self-controlled life by the power of the Holy Spirit who lives in me. I refuse to despise and resist the disciplining of the Lord, which demonstrates His great love for me. I ask this in Jesus' name, amen.

Today we want to look at commitment. Have you ever made a decision during an altar call to repent for overeating and really felt a deep sorrow over it? What happens then when we come up against a temptation and we seem to be bowled over by it? It is in the presence of the Lord that we are deeply touched and feel a desire for repentance. What we need to remember is that we are the temple of the Holy Spirit and carry a portable altar inside of us. The temptation in everyday living can only be met by bringing everything before the presence of the Lord for his strength to meet that temptation. We must learn to acknowledge God in the midst of each circumstance. James 4:6-7 tells us to draw near to God and He will draw near to us. Submit to God, then resist the devil, and he has to flee. When we repent, we are promising to turn towards God's way and away from our own way. We don't have the strength to turn from temptation unless we are turning towards God. In His presence we find the strength to be victorious. Our altar experience needs to become constant. We must be continually in His presence to effect permanent change.

Prayer

Heavenly Father, I thank you for the guidance you provide as a way of escape from my problem by submitting to you. As I acknowledge you in all of my ways I know you will direct my path. Forgive me for trying to do this my own way. Forgive me for leaving you out. Today, I will remember that abiding in you causes me to succeed, and without you I can do nothing. Thank you for bringing me through to an overwhelming victory. As you change me inside, I will lose weight as the outward sign of our deepening relationship. I ask this in Jesus' name, amen.

—Day 12—
He Makes Us Both Willing and Able

Daily Opening Prayer
Heavenly Father, I come to you in the name of my Lord, Jesus Christ to present myself as a living sacrifice, which is my reasonable service. Cleanse me today from the sin of willfulness and fill me with your holiness. Today, I choose to burn the fat on the fire. Accept this offering and enable me to live a self-controlled life by the power of the Holy Spirit who lives in me. I refuse to despise and resist the disciplining of the Lord, which demonstrates His great love for me. I ask this in Jesus' name, amen.

We have previously considered God's instructions from Isaiah 1:19 that told us if we are willing and obedient, we will eat the good of the land. Herein lays the problem. How many times have we known in our hearts what we needed to do, but we just didn't want to? We can make a decision and have good intentions. We start out well, but sooner or later, we get tired of sacrificing and we just quit. We really didn't want to do it in the first place. The good news is that God gave us a way to deal with our **want to**.

The answer, as with everything in our Christian walk, is in Jesus. He is the mediator of a better covenant with better promises. In Philippians 2:13, Paul tells us that God works in us both to will (He gives us the desire to obey) and to do His good pleasure (He gives us the power to do what pleases Him). When we are born again we become new creatures in Christ Jesus. God begins working from the inside out.

God has planted in us, through this new life, a desire to please Him. However, in the beginning, the desire is not strong. Our spirit is willing, but our flesh is not able to be obedient. Because we have been giving in to our appetites, our souls don't have any desire for

41

self-control. This creates conflict between our souls and our spirit. (Read Roman 7).

If we are willing in our spirit to keep making choices that please God and to exercise self control, we will find that an amazing thing happens. We are being inwardly changed while outwardly we are losing weight. Because we are yielding to the Lord, it becomes not a diet, but a deep lifestyle of faith and obedience. He makes us willing and then He makes us able. When we just diet, we are doing sacrifice. What has to happen is that we must present ourselves daily to God as living sacrifices. This is a very hard transition to make. We have to learn to walk in the spirit and not in the flesh. We are making conscious choices to put God in control over and over again. Don't be upset when you realize you have taken the control back. Just repent, submit, and go on. Remember, the blood of Jesus cleanses us continually from all unrighteousness. The key to success is staying submitted. Only God can work this change from the inside out. The decision has to be made that this time I will do this in obedience to the Lord.

As we go along, our bodies losing weight reflect this change outwardly. Again, it is God who is working in us, giving us "the desire to do" and making us "able to do" what pleases Him.

Prayer

Heavenly Father, I thank you for showing me that I don't have to go on struggling to change myself. As I submit to you, you will make me willing and able to please you. Forgive me when I get tired and rebel against this submission. Today, I will not make sacrifices, but will present myself to you as a living sacrifice just as Jesus did. I praise you as I obey your word. You are faithful, encouraging me to want victory and giving me the ability to be victorious. I thank you in Jesus' name, amen.

—Day 13—
Food Is a Problem

Daily Opening Prayer

Heavenly Father, I come to you in the name of my Lord Jesus Christ to present myself as a living sacrifice. I acknowledge this is only my reasonable service. Cleanse me today from the sin of willfulness and fill me with your holiness. Today, I choose to burn the fat on the fire. Accept this offering and enable me to live a self-controlled life by the power of the Holy Spirit who lives in me. I refuse to despise and resist the disciplining of the Lord, which demonstrates His great love for me. I ask this in Jesus name, amen.

From the very beginning of time, mankind eating something when not supposed to has caused problems. The very entrance of sin came through this disobedience of both man and woman. When Adam and Eve chose to eat the forbidden fruit, mankind became aware of sin. Until this time they did not see sin. Evil was present there with them in the garden. Satan was there with all of his corruption. Adam and Eve in their innocence lived freely in the midst of it, but they were unaware of it until by their choice to disobey and eat, their minds were opened. They became aware of good and evil.

Food is something God gave man as a blessing and it is a necessity. Because it immediately gratifies all five senses, Satan has used it to turn a blessing into a curse. Eve listened to him and reached out to take what God had told her not to take. She believed a lie that something good was being withheld from her.

We do the very same thing when we ignore God's Word to us to be temperate and self-controlled. When we ignore these principles long-term it leads to a condition of greed. The definition for "greed" in one part of Webster's dictionary says greed is "a strong desire for food and drink." This is how we form habits. When we begin to practice or exercise temperance and self-control, we will break the bondage of these habits and become conditioned to obedience. Losing weight is our outward result of the inner change.

Remember, immediate gratification feels good up front. We eat a lot of sweets and feel so good until—boom—our blood sugar bottoms out and we hit rock bottom. Isn't this what we've all done? Over and over again we keep choosing quick fixes instead of long-term cures. We need to understand how much God loves us and wants to help us succeed. As we begin to fast ourselves to Him as a living sacrifice (which is what we can do), He will begin to work the changes into our character (which is what He can do). Let's stop struggling and indulging our old natures. Let's begin a new life with Him.

Prayer

Lord, today I acknowledge that I have been living a life of evil self-indulgence. I call it what it is, sin. I repent and ask you to make me able to present myself to you for permanent change. Work in me your desire for self-control, which is a fruit of the Spirit. I will be God—directed and not self-directed. I ask this in Jesus' name, amen.

—Day 14—
Man Shall Not Live by Bread Alone

Daily Opening Prayer

Heavenly Father, I come to you in the name of my Lord, Jesus Christ to present myself as a living sacrifice, which is my reasonable service. Cleanse me today from the sin of willfulness and fill me with your holiness. Today, I choose to burn the fat on the fire. Accept this offering and enable me to live a self-controlled life by the power of the Holy Spirit who lives in me. I refuse to despise and resist the disciplining of the Lord, which demonstrates His great love for me. I ask this in Jesus' name, amen.

Do you often find yourself eating and eating, but never really feeling satisfied? Sometimes the more you eat, the more you want to eat. In Deuteronomy 8:3 we find the words Jesus used against Satan when Satan tempted Him in the wilderness "But He replied, It has been written, Man shall not live and be upheld and sustained by bread alone, but by every word that comes forth from the mouth of God." (Matthew 4:4) The Amplified Bible

We have believed a lie in our souls. We have believed that eating can satisfy our souls' hunger. The reality is that our appetites lie! We buy that lie over and over again, conditioning ourselves to do exactly the opposite thing from what will bring true satisfaction. In Matthew 24:37-39, God warns us that in the end times we are not to be like those in Noah's day—eating and drinking until the flood came and took them all away. Here is a picture of people who continue doing what their flesh wanted them to do. They wouldn't listen to what God was saying to their spirits through Noah. It killed them, folks. They were paying so much attention to their flesh that it dulled their spirits' ability to hear what God was saying.

God is speaking the truth to our spirit and His truth will set us free. We need to grasp the truth of His word when it says, "Man shall not live by bread alone." This truth will help you burn the fat on the fire today and add to your ability to lose weight and keep it off.

Prayer

Heavenly Father, today, I ask you to give me the ability to recognize the true hunger in my life as being a hunger for you. When hunger comes I will begin to fill that hunger with praise, worship, prayer, and meditation. I will eat from your word and deny my flesh. I will defeat the enemy by declaring the word. I will weaken my old fleshly desires by starving them to death. "I know how to live on almost nothing or with everything. I have learned the secret of living in every situation, whether it is with a full stomach or empty, with plenty or little." (Philippians 4:23-24) New Living Translation. Forgive me when I give in and reach for a quick fix. I praise you that as I submit to you I will be changed inside and out. I ask this in Jesus' name, amen.

—Day 15—
Listen to What You Say

Daily Opening Prayer
Heavenly Father, I come to you in the name of my Lord and Savior Jesus Christ to present myself as a living sacrifice, which is my reasonable service. Cleanse me today from the sin of willfulness and fill me with your holiness. Today, I choose to burn the fat on the fire. Accept this offering and enable me to live a self-controlled life by the power of the Holy Spirit who lives in me. I refuse to despise and resist the disciplining of the Lord, which demonstrates His great love for me, amen.

Do you ever look in the mirror and hate the way you look? Do you find yourself making excuses for how you look instead of determining to do something about it? In Matthew 12 Jesus tells us that whatever is in our hearts determines what comes out of our mouths.

Today we are going to look at what kind of confession we have been making. In Proverbs 18 verse 20 and 21 it says that "we have the power of life and death in our mouths." It says words satisfy the soul the same as food satisfies the stomach. In other words, saying the right words brings satisfaction. Whatever you believe in your heart is what comes out of your mouth. You constantly reinforce what you are doing. Let's listen to some confessions.

Do you hear yourself in any of these? "Stockiness runs in my family."

"It doesn't matter what I eat, it all turns to fat anyway."

"I've been really good, I deserve this treat."

"I have diabetes and a metabolic lock, I can't lose weight."

"I've tried dieting; I just can't stick with it."

"My schedule is just too busy, maybe when I finish this project I'll be able to do it."

"I'll just have one more helping; it won't hurt just this once." And this seems to be a favorite: "I don't do anything else wrong; eating isn't as bad as stealing or lying." Or how about, "I eat less than people who are thin and I'm still fat." What we say determines what we will do; what we do forms habits and shapes our lifestyle.

Let's go right to the heart of the matter and begin to listen to what we are saying. How can we change our negative confessions into positive ones? The answer is simple. We can't. God has to change us. Our part is to stop focusing on the outward appearance and announcing all of the excuses for why it's okay to fail. Let's begin to do the word and present ourselves to God as living sacrifices, allowing Him to transform us by the renewing of our minds. When we meditate on and confess the negative, we are eating death. When we meditate on and confess God's Word, we are eating from life. As we speak the Word, we are feeding our inner man. We are making our spirits fat, not our bodies.

The Bible says in Philippians 4:13, "I can do all things through Christ who strengthens me." We read in Mark 10 verse 27 that all things are possible if we only believe. Our part is to believe God's Word is true. Begin to read your Bible and as you do ask the Holy Spirit to help you find your own positive confessions. As you are changed on the inside, your outward habits will be changed. You will lose weight as a natural consequence.

Prayer

Heavenly Father, I thank you that you have made a way to escape for me out of my lifestyle of death. I acknowledge that my confession has been negative and has led me to fail. Forgive me. Today, I believe you are changing my heart, my confession, and my lifestyle. This will cause me to lose weight as a direct result of this inward change. Psalm 19:14 says, "Let the words of my mouth, and the meditation of my heart, be acceptable in Thy sight, O LORD, my strength, and my redeemer." (King James Version) I ask this in Jesus' name, amen.

—Day 16—
No Flesh Will Glory in His Presence

Daily Opening Prayer
Heavenly Father, I come to you in the name of my Lord, Jesus Christ to present myself as a living sacrifice, which is my reasonable service. Cleanse me today from the sin of willfulness and fill me with your holiness. Today, I choose to burn the fat on the fire. Accept this offering and enable me to live a self-controlled life by the power of the Holy Spirit who lives in me. I refuse to despise and resist the disciplining of the Lord, which demonstrates His great love for me. I ask this in Jesus' name, amen.

How many times do we go through expensive and timely preparations so that we look "just right?" Being overweight makes this even harder because what we see in the mirror is not pleasing to our eyes. Today people in general seem to have only the outward appearance on their minds. In 1 Corinthians 7:31 Paul reminds us that the fashion of this world is passing away. God wants to move into the area of our life that is controlling these fleshly desires. He wants to show us how empty they really are. In his second letter to the Corinthians, Paul reminds them that everything they can see is temporary. He tells them that what they can't see is eternal (2 Corinthians 4:18). The very way God chooses to work disallows any boasting on man's part. First Corinthians 1:28-29 tells us that God's intention is that no flesh will ever be able to glory in His presence. As we said before, God works from the inside out.

The method He has chosen to demonstrate His mighty power takes us right back to the cross. We identify with Christ when He was crucified that this power is released. That is why Paul tells us in Romans 12 to present ourselves to God as living sacrifices, which is only our reasonable service. It's only what we're supposed to be doing. As we say no to being controlled by temporary pleasures that feed our egos and our bodies and begin to say yes to the discipline that denies our flesh, we open the door to this divine power. It will change us. A miracle begins to work within us. Every inner work of God will have an outward demonstration. In our case, as the flesh dies from our inner man, weight is lost from our bodies on the outside. We will never be able to boast that we did this because we made it happen. We are called to only boast about what God has done for us and in us (1 Corinthians 1:31).

Prayer

Heavenly Father, I thank you for showing me how shallow my preoccupation with outward appearance really is. Forgive me when I allow outward influences to gain control of my focus, and I stop looking to you for my answers. Forgive me for making temporary things more important than eternal ones. Help me remember that no flesh will glory in your presence. Today, I will present myself as a living sacrifice which will allow your mighty power to work change in me. I praise you and thank You for this miracle, which is manifested in my body. We thank you in Jesus' name, amen.

—Day 17—
We Build Shrines That Become Prisons

Daily Opening Prayer
Heavenly Father, I come to you in the name of my Lord, Jesus Christ to present myself as a living sacrifice, which is my reasonable service. Cleanse me today from the sin of willfulness and fill me with your holiness. Today, I choose to burn the fat on the fire. Accept this offering and enable me to live a self-controlled life by the power of the Holy Spirit who lives in me. I refuse to despise and resist the disciplining of the Lord, which demonstrates His great love for me. I ask this in Jesus' name, amen.

How often do we have the sense that there are iron bars built all around us? The truth is we have built ourselves into prisons. The lie is that there is no key to let us out. In fact, sometimes it seems like there isn't even a door. Jesus said that He was the Door (John 10: 7). In Revelation 3:8 we are told that God has set before us an open door that no man can shut. In 1 Corinthians 16:9 Paul was given a great and effective open door. Jesus said in Luke 4:18 that He had come to set captives free. God is no respecter of persons. There is absolutely no prison that Jesus cannot walk into. Once there, He Himself is our doorway out. And how do we get into these prisons? Anything we allow to become more important than the Lord becomes an idol. As we habitually worship these idols, we are actually building a shrine around them. We have made many things into idols. Money, our children, our positions, our Christian service, and for those of us who are overweight—food. We worship at this shrine daily. Over and over again, we seek this part of God's creation rather than the Creator, Himself.

John warns us as little children to guard ourselves from idols (1 John 5:21). Each time we choose to serve our fleshly appetites we strengthen this shrine. We must see that by making these choices we allow the enemy a way to ensnare us. We don't realize we've been building a shrine for our food idols until we find ourselves trapped, wondering, *how did this happen?* Suddenly we are in a prison that doesn't seem to have a door.

Deliverance will only come when we cry out to Jesus for help. He has actually been with us the whole time. Because our attention has been focused on gratifying our fleshly desires, we haven't seen Him! God has allowed the misery of this imprisonment to become so painful we finally turned our eyes upon Jesus with the determination to follow Him out. As we do this the shrine dissolves. The Lord Himself replaces the idols of food. We see the truth that the only way to stay free is to make Jesus the center of our existence. This will be a step-by-step walking out as we continually choose to keep our focus on Him.

Prayer

Heavenly Father, I thank you for providing Jesus as the way out of the prison of lies my self-indulgent choices have built. Forgive me for ignoring you and focusing on my own fleshly desires. Today, I choose to keep my eyes fixed on Jesus as He leads me out of this bondage. I praise you and thank You that as I continue to do this, my soul is set free from sin and my body will be set free from fat. I ask this in Jesus' name, amen.

—Day 18—
No Condemnation

Daily Opening Prayer

Heavenly Father, I come to you in the name of my Lord, Jesus Christ to present myself as a living sacrifice, which is my reasonable service. Cleanse me today from the sin of willfulness and fill me with your holiness. Today, I choose to burn the fat on the fire. Accept this offering and enable me to live a self-controlled life by the power of the Holy Spirit who lives in me. I refuse to despise and resist the disciplining of the Lord, which demonstrates His great love for me. I ask this in Jesus' name, amen.

In Romans 8 we read that there is **now** no condemnation to those who are in Christ Jesus. These are truly wonderful words! Do we really understand what they mean to us in our everyday life? Going back to Romans 8 we read how the power of the life-giving Spirit has set us free. Through Jesus Christ, the power of sin that leads to death has been broken.

When we continue to live a life of immediate gratification, it keeps leading us back to failure over and over again. Our minds tell us what total losers we are and not of weight! We go on overeating, gaining more weight on our bodies, and living under a horrible sense of being condemned to this kind of lifestyle forever. This is a lie!

God has prepared a way to escape for us in the midst of this temptation. If we can by faith put ourselves into Jesus Christ, we die to ourselves and become alive to God. It can be compared to a pregnant woman who is at the point of delivery. She has experienced labor pains, but suddenly they take over. No longer is she pushing and trying to bear down. She is caught up in a process that is greater than she is. The woman is no longer afraid of this process of delivery.

She feels herself being pulled into something she knows will bring her to a glorious end. The delivery of a new life!

The Bible tells us in Colossians that through faith in the operation of God we are raised from death into life. This can be compared to the way a woman is caught up in the labor and delivery process. The key in both situations is surrendering to the process. At this point we are set free. Spiritually speaking, we enter into the death of Jesus Christ experientially. It is at this point that we become alive to God.

When someone is dead, there is no way for the temptations in the world to bother them any longer. The dead person is just that, dead. This includes being dead to condemnation. When we surrender to the operation of God, it is the point where we undergo death to self. As we die to self, we become alive to God and are then made able by the Holy Spirit, who lives in us, to experience this new life.

This is not giving us a license to live any way we choose. Rather, we are given the liberty to choose God's way, free of condemnation and able to make wise choices. This will lead to permanent inner change as we exercise those right choices over and over again. Our weight loss is the natural outward manifestation of our new inward freedom. We can now live relaxed and victorious lives.

Prayer

Heavenly Father, I thank you for providing a way to escape from living under the sense of failure that brings condemnation. I know that in Jesus Christ I have been set free to live a life of liberty and success. I confess that I have tried to win this victory on my own and have failed miserably. Today, I surrender and submit to you by faith. In the midst of the onslaught of the enemy and my own old nature, I refuse to recognize the battle. I reckon myself dead to sin and alive to you. Thank You for giving me the victory and a new way of living. Thank You for permanent inner change, which will lead to permanent weight loss. I ask this in Jesus' name, amen.

—Day 19—

Cause Me to Remember

Daily Opening Prayer

Heavenly Father, I come to you in the name of my Lord, Jesus Christ to present myself as a living sacrifice, which is my reasonable service. Cleanse me today from the sin of willfulness and fill me with your holiness. Today, I choose to burn the fat on the fire. Accept this offering and enable me to live a self-controlled life by the power of the Holy Spirit who lives in me. I refuse to despise and resist the disciplining of the Lord, which demonstrates His great love for me. I ask this in Jesus' name, amen.

Memories can be wonderful, awful, stimulating, depressing; they can bring joy and sometimes sorrow. We all have them, and they affect us according to our own personalities. At one place in God's Word we are counseled to forget those things that are behind and press on. In other parts of the Bible we are exhorted to remember. Is the scripture contradictory here? No, the instructions to forget what is behind simply means don't get sidetracked by past incidents. We must not allow events from our past to hold us back from pressing on towards the future God has planned for us. When we are exhorted to remember, it is so that we can clearly see how faithful God has always been. We recall the times that we have been weak and His strength has brought us through.

Each time we walk through tribulation and testing we gain in three areas of our lives. First, inwardly, these times perfect our faith and cause it to grow stronger (1 Peter 1:6-9). We are encouraged each time we see God's Word manifested in our lives. We build a foundation layer-by-layer that is based on God's faithfulness to us no matter what we are facing. This foundation is unshakable and will stand eternally.

Secondly, we are being conformed to the image of Jesus Christ (Romans 8: 29). We gain compassion as we remember our helplessness and inability to end our struggle ourselves; the answer is always Jesus Christ (Romans 7:24-25). As our high priest, Jesus is touched by the feeling of our infirmities. In every way the things that tempt us also tempted Him. The difference is He never yielded. As part of His body, we must be able not only to receive His victory, but remember that He struggled, too.

Lastly, we gain the outward answer. Let us remember our struggle to lose weight and how helpless and hopeless it sometimes seems. Let us remember being sick at heart until we began to see God's wonderful love as He identified with us in the midst of the struggle. It is in this time of testing that we are able to gain a new compassion for others. We are allowed the privilege of helping someone else because we know exactly what he or she is going through. All of this produces a permanent inner change, which then causes our bodies to conform. Our weight loss becomes the natural result of our being spiritually aligned with God's purpose for our lives.

Prayer

Heavenly Father, I thank you for the memories that make me able to see your faithfulness in every situation. Forgive me for the times I forget it is only your grace to me that gives the victory and not my own way of doing things. It is your gift and not my own efforts that will bring permanent change and weight loss. Today, I will forget the failures that have kept me from trying. I will remember you in the midst of each temptation and you will bring me through. I praise your holy name, amen.

—Day 20—
Valuing Yourself God's Way

Daily Opening Prayer
Heavenly Father, I come to you in the name of my Lord, Jesus Christ to present myself as a living sacrifice, which is my reasonable service. Cleanse me today from the sin of willfulness and fill me with your holiness. Today, I choose to burn the fat on the fire. Accept this offering and enable me to live a self-controlled life by the power of the Holy Spirit who lives in me. I refuse to despise and resist the disciplining of the Lord, which demonstrates His great love for me. I ask this in Jesus' name, amen.

Every human being is born with a God-given need for a sense of worth and purpose. If you're like the majority of overweight people who have fought the "fat battle" most of their lives, it has left you feeling totally worthless. You have no purpose except just to survive. The trouble here is that man has put the emphasis totally on the outward appearance. When we try to handle the overweight problem, we have been pre-programmed to work on the outside, leaving our inside completely untouched.

Hollywood, the media, advertising, everything around us says, "If you're fat, you are a loser." When we do have a temporary victory and gain a semblance of outward thinness we find it an empty victory. The things that were hurting us have not been healed. We live in bondage and misery to the fear of gaining the weight back. Most of the time, we do gain it back.

God knows that permanent weight loss must begin on the inside. He wants us to see this truth and be set free forever. Roman 5: 6 teaches us that when we were utterly helpless, Christ came at just the right time and died for us sinners. This is the value that God has placed on us. He loves us so much that He gave the best heaven had to offer, His only Son! Once we begin to understand that God values us at our worst, we can relax and realize we don't change so God will love us more. We change because He loves us so much! We realize He cares about us the way we are. This sets us free to be obedient, because we want to, not because we have to. We begin to understand that His instructions to us lead to a healthier, happier life while we are here on Earth. He does not require rigid rules to make us more acceptable. We have once and for all time been made acceptable in the Beloved: through the death, burial, and resurrection of our brother, Jesus.

Prayer

Heavenly Father, thank you that you love me just the way I am. Help me to receive this love and relax in it. Forgive me when I forget and think I have to change myself to become more acceptable to you. I praise you that I am fearfully and wonderfully made. I am loved right where I am. Today, I will remember how much you value me. I will submit to you, resist the enemy when he tries to tell me I am worthless, and be changed in my inner man through this process. I will lose weight as an outward sign of my inner obedience. I ask this in Jesus' name, amen.

—Day 21—
Be a Doer of the Word

Daily Opening Prayer
Heavenly Father, I come to you in the name of my Lord, Jesus Christ to present myself as a living sacrifice, which is my reasonable service. Cleanse me today from the sin of willfulness and fill me with your holiness. Today, I choose to burn the fat on the fire. Accept this offering and enable me to live a self-controlled life by the power of the Holy Spirit who lives in me. I refuse to despise and resist the disciplining of the Lord, which demonstrates His great love for me. I ask in Jesus' name, amen.

In James 1:21-23 we are told to get rid of evil things in our lives. We are to humbly accept and obey God's message to us from His word. We are cautioned to remember that hearing is not enough. The message must be obeyed. In all of God's instruction to us, there are always two parts; our part and His part. James is telling us that if we receive God's Word and obey it, the Word itself is alive and will change us (save us). We will be blessed if we don't forget.

Second Peter 1 promises us that everything we need for living a godly life is ours by getting to know Jesus better. Through these promises God's divine power makes His own nature available to us. Then we will no longer live according to the dictates of our flesh. Peter encouraged believers to make every effort to apply these promises to their lives.

When we believe and do these promises, our faith produces a life of moral excellence. The definition of moral excellence means being strong in doing what is right. As we do what God shows us in His word, we get to know Him better. When we know Him better it leads to self-control. Self-control allows us to patiently endure when we are tried and tested. Patient endurance begins producing God's own nature inside of us. And finally, all of this leads to brotherly kindness. We will have God and love in our hearts. This makes us able to be productive and useful with what we have learned.

Remember, if we fail to develop these virtues, Peter tells us we are blind and shortsighted. We keep forgetting that God has cleansed us from our old life of sin through the blood of His Son. God wants to set his people free from the destructive force of overeating. When we realize this and begin applying His word of moderation to outward eating habits, we will get to know Him better. Knowing Him better allows Him to produce His character in us.

When we are willing to go through this process we are set free from our bondage to food. If we don't put into practice what we know to be His instruction, we are in sin. This sin keeps us in the prison our fleshly habits have created. It prevents God from liberating us. We must become hearers and doers of the Word.

Prayer

Heavenly Father, I thank you for your word that is truth. Forgive me that I have not always put what I hear into action. Today, I will do my part so you can do your part. I will moderate my eating habits as you are at work inside me giving me the power I need to succeed and be changed. I praise you and thank you for setting me free. I ask this in Jesus' name, amen.

—Day 22—

Let Your Moderation Be Known

Daily Opening Prayer

Heavenly Father, I come to you in the name of my Lord, Jesus Christ to present myself as a living sacrifice, which is my reasonable service. Cleanse me today from the sin of willfulness and fill me with your holiness. Today, I choose to burn the fat on the fire. Accept this offering and enable me to live a self-controlled life by the power of the Holy Spirit who lives in me. I refuse to despise and resist the disciplining of the Lord, which demonstrates His great love for me. I ask this in Jesus' name, amen.

We are all aware of the pace in the world around us. We are programmed to want faster everything: faster communications, faster internet service, faster travel, fast food, fast cars, and faster results with diet and exercise. A lot of money is spent in a quest for these things. The problem is: easy come—easy go.

In Philippians 4:5 Paul instructs us to let our moderation be known to all men. He also gave us the reason for this; the Lord is at hand. In Isaiah 18 God calls us to come to Him and reason together. He tells us here that if we will obey Him we will always have plenty to eat.

Because we are living in the last days, the enemy of our souls has only one goal, our destruction. He is constantly whipping mankind into a state of frenzied activity. He wants no time left for reasonable consideration. The prophet tells the people, in Isaiah 30:15, that in returning to God and resting in Him, they would be saved. In His quietness and confidence will be their strength. God has always called his people out from the ways of the world. In Proverbs 16:25 we read there is a way that seems right to mankind, but the end of that way leads to death. When we get caught up in today's whirlwind lifestyle, we cut ourselves off from God's help. We must make a conscious decision to step aside from the rat race. Through this study of the Word and prayer we come to know God and His ways. As we walk in His ways, He can change us. "All scripture is inspired by God and is useful to teach us what is true and to make us realize what is wrong in our lives. It straightens us out and teaches us to do what is right. It is God's way of preparing us in every way, fully equipped for every good thing God wants us to do." (2 Timothy 3:16-17) New Living Translation

When we choose to exercise moderation, our minds become unclouded from all the worldly cares that distract us. We are changed and become able to hear and do the Word. As we seek the Lord first, whichever weight loss program we choose becomes easier to follow. We need to be responsible and choose to follow a healthy plan. We can reject the lure of quick fixes that don't last anyway. We can settle into God's perfect pace for us individually. When our minds and our spirits are in agreement, our bodies have to come along. When our minds are at enmity against God, we want to do our own thing and it always leaves God out. We cheat ourselves from being able to have God's best when we supply ourselves with what we can do. It is with a moderate lifestyle that we can fully experience God's help right now.

Prayer

Heavenly Father, thank you for the rest and quietness you provide in Jesus Christ. Forgive me when I let the cares of this world distract me. Forgive me when I allow myself to become a part of the rat race. Today, I will exercise moderation. I will read your word and be instructed by you. I thank you and praise you that as I choose your ways your helps are immediately available to me. My victory is assured because of your faithfulness. I ask this in Jesus' name, amen.

—Day 23—
Patient Endurance

Daily Opening Prayer

Heavenly Father, I come to you in the name of my Lord, Jesus Christ to present myself as a living sacrifice, which is my reasonable service. Cleanse me today from the sin of willfulness and fill me with your holiness. Today, I choose to burn the fat on the fire. Accept this offering and enable me to live a self-controlled life by the power of the Holy Spirit who lives in me. I refuse to despise and resist the disciplining of the Lord, which demonstrates His great love for me. I ask this in Jesus' name, amen.

For most of us, enduring a weight loss program to the end has been a very difficult thing to do. We can feel cheated, starved, and foolish for even trying. Many times we are defeated before we ever get started. None of this leads to the kind of lasting success we are longing for. When we begin a weight loss program, the results are what we are looking for. And we want them right now! Here again, we need to consider our motive. It needs to be obedience and a desire to please the Lord more than a daily pound loss and looking good.

In Hebrews 12:1-2 we are instructed (see the humor here) to lay aside every weight and the sin that so easily besets us and run with patience the course that is set before us. We are told to look to Jesus, not results in our outward appearance, because He is the author and finisher of our faith. In Hebrews 11 we are told what faith is. It is the confident assurance that what we hope for is going to happen. That means it is already ours. It is the evidence of things we cannot yet see.

For most of us weight loss is not a sprint that will be over in a short time. It is a marathon that requires us to find a pace we can endure. We have to run this race until we cross the finish line. This is where patient endurance comes in. The good part of this exercise is we are not actually running a physical race. This is something a lot of us don't like to do anyway.

Our exercise is spiritual and it produces strength in our inner man. It causes strength to be infused into us directly from Jesus. We have to realize here that we are **not** fighting against physical, outward weaknesses. We are fighting a fight of faith. It is through this fight that we enter into the faith of Jesus Himself. We don't need to be afraid of getting to the end of our own strength, because it is in our weakness that His strength is made perfect. God is always faithful to His Word. If we choose His way, we will succeed.

Galatians 6:9 tells us not to grow weary in well doing for in due season we shall reap if we faint not. Hebrews 12:3 says that we first faint in our minds. We are crucified with Christ, but live this life in the flesh by the faith of the Son of God who loves us and gave Himself for us (Galatians 2:20). Therefore, we only need to go on exercising the patience God gives us. It will grow stronger as we do this and the end result will be the inward change we are looking for. This will produce change in our outward appearance through weight loss. Doing things God's way always works best and produces eternal results.

Prayer

Heavenly Father, I confess I have been trying to run this race in my own strength. I have always failed. Forgive me. I will begin today to run this race keeping my eyes on Jesus and allowing His faith to become mine. I know as I choose your ways I cannot fail. Thank you for changing me inside so my outward weight loss happens as a direct result of my patient endurance. I will run this race and win. Your word says I can. Praise you for your wonderful plan, which always gives me the best and not what I would settle for. I ask this in Jesus' name, amen.

—Day 24—
God's Daily Provision

Daily Opening Prayer

Heavenly Father, I come to you in the name of my Lord, Jesus Christ to present myself as a living sacrifice, which is my reasonable service. Cleanse me today from the sin of willfulness and fill me with your holiness. Today, I choose to burn the fat on the fire. Accept this offering and enable me to live a self-controlled life by the power of the Holy Spirit who lives in me. I refuse to despise and resist the disciplining of the Lord, which demonstrates His great love for me. I ask this in Jesus' name, amen.

God created each one of us with a measure of faith. In Hebrews 11:6 we are told that without faith it is impossible to please God. Since we were created for His pleasure, it would seem faith is the way that we do this. The Bible says we must come to God believing that He is and that He rewards of those who diligently seek Him. Again, faith allows us to do this. How we live our lives on a daily basis and the choices we make either strengthen or weaken our faith.

We are taught that we must fight the good fight of faith. It seems that faith is the thread that weaves us into either a strong tapestry for God to use, or the lack of it makes us a weak cloth full of tears and holes. We are not fit for much of anything useful that way.

Let's consider how to exercise our faith so it becomes strong and powerful. It is God's gift to us for a successful existence here on this earth. Faith is like a muscle which grows stronger as we exercise it. Actually, it is more like a trained response. When an athlete does the same thing over and over again it becomes an automatic action. The signals in the nervous system get so conditioned there is a continual unbroken flow in the exercise. We call this coordination. The same thing can happen with the measure of faith God has given us. When we choose to put all of our faith into Jesus Christ, He makes His perfect faith available to us. We must repeat this process over and over again until it becomes part of our nature.

Many years ago, Dr. David Goodwin, founder of Christian Life Worship Center, in Des Moines Iowa, taught a series on "The Faith of Christ". He pointed out that the only faith that can please God is the perfect faith of His Son. As we totally submit to the Lord and allow Him to live His life through us, He makes us able to live by Jesus' own faith. This and this alone pleases God. It is as we consider ourselves dead to sin we become able to live (Romans 6:11). Paul sums it up in Galatians 2:15 when he says that through the law of God we are made aware of our inability to please God.

We must practice this truth in the area of weight control until it becomes an automatic response. It is not exercising our own faith, but living this life in the flesh by the faith of the Son of God who loves us and gave Himself for us that gives us victory. We are thrust into Jesus' power and entered into His fulfillment of the law.

Prayer

Heavenly Father, I thank you that in Jesus Christ you have made a way for me to please you. Forgive me when I put faith in my own efforts and not in what He has already accomplished. Today, I will access His perfect faith, which will make me able to overcome the fleshly appetites that have kept me in bondage and failure. I praise you and thank you that through this process my victory is assured. I will lose weight as an outward sign of my inner choices. I ask this in Jesus' name amen.

—Day 25—
Breaking Free—Do Not Despise
the Discipline

Daily Opening Prayer

Heavenly Father, I come to you in the name of my Lord, Jesus Christ to present myself as a living sacrifice, which is my reasonable service. Cleanse me today from the sin of willfulness and fill me with your holiness. Today, I choose to burn the fat on the fire. Accept this offering and enable me to live a self-controlled life by the power of the Holy Spirit who lives in me. I refuse to despise and resist the disciplining of the Lord, which demonstrates His great love for me. I ask this in Jesus' name, amen.

Have you gone through a diet regimen only to be relieved when it was over? You reached your outward goal, you look good, but no change has actually taken place inside. Within weeks or months you find yourself slipping back into your old habits and gaining the weight back. All of this happens, because we despise the discipline of the diet. We tolerate it just long enough to reach our goal; then, we gradually go back to overeating because we truly hate the process.

There are three steps to breaking free from this pattern.

We must acknowledge and receive the truth that the amount we eat and the choices we make are why we are overweight. We can't continue to eat this way and have permanent weight loss. The world is now offering ways to continue doing the wrong things without suffering the consequences. We can use carbohydrate blockers, fat blockers, starvation diets, diet pills, diet drinks, and any number of other quick fixes. These programs all offer us a way to change our outward appearance. The only change that lasts will come from His discipline that instructs and corrects the inward man.

We must be willing to receive the instruction and correction necessary to bring about a permanent change in the way we think about food. There's an old saying: "You live to eat or you eat to live." Which category describes your thinking? The only discipline God imposed on Adam and Eve in the Garden of Eden was not to eat from the Tree of the Knowledge of Good and Evil. He told them that for their own good. God made man able to eat as a pleasurable way of satisfying his physical needs. Lust caused man to take more than he needed, and we are still doing it today. God intended food as a blessing, man's choices turned into a curse.

We must realize and acknowledge that the only way to real freedom is through Jesus Christ. Jesus totally identified with us in our inability to trust God. Though he was tempted by the devil to choose a quick fix after his 40-day fast in the desert, He refused. He willingly denied Himself so that He was acceptable to God as the perfect sacrifice for all sin. Our sin of overeating was nailed to the cross with Him. As we identify with Him in this living sacrificial death, we are set free. We are then raised from living in death to walking in newness of life. John 8:36 says whom the Son sets free is free indeed.

Finally, when we understand the love of God we are made able to receive His correction and instruction with joy. Understanding God's way of disciplining will cause us to see discipline as a good thing, given for our benefit.

Prayer
Heavenly Father, forgive me for despising your discipline, correction, and instruction for my life. Cause me to understand the benefit in following Your way. Today, I choose to acknowledge you in all my ways. I will not lean unto my own understanding. I willingly submit to your loving discipline calling it a good thing. As I do this, you will continually set me free. I praise you for your faithfulness to me through Jesus Christ, my Lord, amen.

—Day 26—
Acknowledge Sin

Daily Opening Prayer
Heavenly Father, I come to you in the name of my Lord, Jesus Christ to present myself as a living sacrifice, which is my reasonable service. Cleanse me today from the sin of willfulness and fill me with your holiness. Today, I choose to burn the fat on the fire. Accept this offering and enable me to live a self-controlled life by the power of the Holy Spirit who lives in me. I refuse to despise and resist the disciplining of the Lord, which demonstrates His great love for me. I ask this in Jesus' name, amen.

In today's world we are given every excuse man's mind can think of to get out of being responsible for our actions. However, any excuse we make to call the sin in our lives by any other name does not negate the facts. It is still sin. When we live our lives in the flesh, directed by the world working through our old nature, we are in sin!

In Romans 5:20 The Bible tells us in Romans 5: 2 that God's law was given so all people could see how sinful they really are. Acknowledging sin in our lives is the first step toward being set free from it. Until we do this, most of our overweight conditions are a direct result of sinful choices. We are bound by the lie that we are helpless in the midst of this. Victim mentality makes us resentful, even of the Lord. Because we are locked into this cycle of sinning, we constantly beg forgiveness and feel condemned. This is **not** God's plan for our lives.

Not only are we forgiven in Christ Jesus, but also the power of sin is broken over our lives. Romans 7:6 read as follows, "But now we have been released from the law, for we died with Christ, and we are no longer captive to its power. Now we can really serve God, not in the old way by obeying the letter of the law, but in the new way, by the Spirit." (New Living Translation)

Romans 6:18 tells us that we have been set free from our old master of sin, so we can now serve our new Master in righteousness. This means we are free to choose by faith those things that will please God. Rather than continuing to stuff our bodies with food, let each bite we take be to the glory of God.

Prayer

Heavenly Father, I thank you for helping me to acknowledge sin in my life. By looking into your perfect law, I am able to see the truth. Forgive me for blaming my overweight problem on excuses and allowing a root of bitterness to grow in my heart. Today, I call the choices I make to indulge my flesh as sin. I repent and ask you to forgive me. I praise and thank you that you have given me the power of your truth. Your word is setting me free. The root of bitterness will die as I continue to accept responsibility for my eating habits. I praise you and thank You that I choose to obey you because I want to and not because I have to. I ask this in Jesus' name, amen.

—Day 27—
Gluttony

Daily Opening Prayer

Heavenly Father, I come to you in the name of my Lord, Jesus Christ to present myself as a living sacrifice, which is my reasonable service. Cleanse me today from the sin of willfulness and fill me with your holiness. Today, I choose to burn the fat on the fire. Accept this offering and enable me to live a self-controlled life by the power of the Holy Spirit who lives in me. I refuse to despise and resist the disciplining of the Lord, which demonstrates His great love for me. I ask this in Jesus' name, amen.

Habitual overeating leads to becoming a glutton. The dictionary root word for glutton is glut, which means the supply exceeds the demand. A glutton is a person who eats to excess. Gluttony means the habit of eating too much. Once we have formed habits, we lose control and eating becomes compulsive. Are you able to eat a measured portion, or do you all of a sudden find yourself eating until the container is empty? Do you say to yourself, *I only meant to have a few bites—what happened?*

Mike Murdock, wisdom teacher and songwriter, teaches that we determine our habits and our habits determine our futures. In Romans 14:17 Paul tells us that the Kingdom of God is not meat or drink (temporal things); but righteousness, peace and joy in the Holy Ghost. Let's ask ourselves, *are we serving our appetites or are we serving the Lord?* Have our habits trapped us into making the wrong choices over and over until we feel hopeless and condemned? Many Christians say, "I've done everything and nothing has helped, it's not my fault." The good news is that Jesus Christ came not only to forgive us for sin, but He came to break the power of sin over our lives. Read Romans 7 where Paul describes the struggle to put your own specific struggle with compulsive overeating into it. It is only through Jesus Christ, who is the Way, the Truth, and the Life, that we are set free.

Prayer

Heavenly Father, I admit to you that I have lost control. I confess the sin of gluttony and I repent. I believe I am forgiven, and you are breaking the power of the sin over my life. Today, I will yield to You, Holy Spirit, so you can make me able to choose self control and not give into my old appetites. I thank you that as I do this, you will give me the ability to make wise choices in my eating habits. I ask this in Jesus' name, amen.

—Day 28—
Whose God Is Their Belly

Daily Opening Prayer

Heavenly Father, I come to you in the name of my Lord and Savior Jesus Christ to offer myself as a living sacrifice, which is my reasonable service. Cleanse me today from the sin of willfulness and fill me with your holiness. Today, I choose to burn the fat on the fire. Accept this offering and enable me to live a self-controlled life by the power of the Holy Spirit who us in me. I refuse to despise and resist the disciplining of the Lord, which demonstrates His great love for me. I ask this in Jesus' name, amen.

(Read Philippians 4:17-21) Paul was grieving over the peoples' misconduct showing them as enemies of the cross of Christ. He pointed out several problems in their lives, especially referring to the fact that they only thought about things of this earth. He said their God was their belly (appetites). We know that he was talking about all fleshly appetites, but for our purposes, we will look at it from the problem of overeating.

Do you find yourself being controlled by what your belly demands? Romans 6:16 says, "Know ye not, that to whom ye yield yourself servants to obey, his servants ye are to whom you obey; whether of sin unto death, or of obedience unto righteousness?" (King James Version) If we are being controlled by our desire to overeat, then we are in bondage to that desire. We cannot live in the liberty that Christ purchased for us if we are continuing in bondage to our belly's demand to be fed. Remember, if we are servants to sin, it leads to death.

The sin of overeating separates us from God's best. It affects our relationship with Him. It even causes problems in our relationships with each other. It also brings about natural consequences: health problems, both physical and psychological. The result of overeating that ends in death is one of Satan's greatest victories over us. How in the world can we break free?

As we continue in Romans 6:17 Paul says, "Thank God! Once you were slaves of sin, but now you have obeyed with all your heart the new teaching God has given you. Now you are free from sin, your old master, and you have become slaves to your new master, righteousness." (New Living Translation) As we deny ourselves and our old fleshly appetites, they grow weaker through practicing obedience and discipline. God changes our desires and makes us able to live more and more in His perfect plan for our lives. Jesus truly sets us free.

Prayer

Heavenly Father, I confess I have been the servant to my appetites. Forgive me and restore me into the liberty that is mine in Jesus Christ. I will yield myself to obey you from my heart. Thank you for changing me and causing me to begin to live and not die. The Holy Spirit helps me today to keep on making the right choices. I praise you that as I do these things, I will be changed inside and out. Weight loss will be to your glory and not to please my ego. I ask this in Jesus' name, amen.

—Day 29—
Eating the Good of the Land

Daily Opening Prayer
Heavenly Father, I come to you in name of my Lord and Savior Jesus Christ to present myself as a living sacrifice, which is my reasonable service. Cleanse me today from the sin of willfulness and fill me with your holiness. Today, I choose to burn the fat on the fire. Accept this offering and enable me to live a self-controlled life by the power of the Holy Spirit who lives in me. I refuse to despise and resist the disciplining of the Lord, which demonstrates His great love for me, amen.

We are taught that if we are willing to hear and be obedient we will eat the good of the land. "If you will only obey me and let me help you, then you will have plenty to eat." (Isaiah 1: 19) New Living Translation When we live in fear and greed, nothing satisfies the basic inner need we have to be filled. We are afraid that we aren't ever going to have enough to eat. God created us with a need to eat in order to live. Today's world has sold people a lie. What they call "good food" is basically food with no nutritional value. We are bombarded with commercials showing every way possible to get something fast. Let's coin a new phrase. **Fast Makes Fat!** Why is it we are in such a rush? What is it we are hurrying so fast to get to?

Our bodies have a need to be satisfied with proper, nourishing foods. When we resort to the quick fix answers, we cheat our bodies out of the ability to rebuild them and maintain optimum health. The end result is a constantly hungry existence. God also made food to be a delight to the soul. He even promises that one of our first experiences in Heaven will be sitting down at a banquet table.

As we constantly provide ourselves with the easy fast food answers, we are also feeding our fleshly inner man and making him in charge. This affects every part of our lives. We want everything right now!

In the Garden of Eden, Satan used the same lie we are being told today. He said, "Here's a fast food way to satisfy your real inner hunger. Eat the fruit and become like God." This is where things were turned upside down. We must see that we have to first become willing to do things God's way. When we become willing, we must then put action to our willingness and become obedient. Again, God works from the inside out.

God, from the beginning of time, provided food for the body and Himself for the soul. Even Jesus said, "I am the Bread of Life." When God says He wants us to eat "the good of the land," He means He wants us to have the very best there is to offer. Our problem seems to be in thinking that what's best is what's most convenient. We want no effort on our part. We have to see the truth. What sometimes seems most convenient and effortless leaves us unsatisfied with the demand for more.

The only answer is when we acknowledge our need to present ourselves to God as living sacrifices, and allow Him to transform us by the renewing of our minds. We must believe that He cares about our need to be satisfied. (Read Romans 12:1-2.)

Let's stop depending on diets and programs that cost a fortune, promise a quick result, but never bring us into that good land where we are permanently changed. Let us begin to "eat the good of the land" and be eternally satisfied. If we choose God's way, we'll be OK!

Prayer

Heavenly Father, I thank you, Lord, for making me willing to stop choosing quick fix answers. Forgive me when I fail to see your way is best. Today, I choose to believe you will lead me to eat right and be completely satisfied inside and out. As I listen to you and do what you tell me I will begin to walk in this new land of health and happiness. You will nourish my soul with yourself and my body with good food. Thank you again, for your love and provision, which is always perfect. I ask this in Jesus' name, amen.

—Day 30—

You May Be out of Egypt, but Is Egypt out of You?

Daily Opening Prayer
Heavenly Father, I come to you in the name of my Lord and Savior, Jesus Christ, to present myself as a living sacrifice, which is my reasonable service. Cleanse me today from the sin of willfulness and fill me with your holiness. Today, I choose to burn the fat on the fire. Accept this offering and enable me to live a self-controlled life by the power of the Holy Spirit who lives in me. I refuse to despise and resist the disciplining of the Lord, which demonstrates His great love for me. I ask this in Jesus' name, amen.

Almost everyone, whether a Christian or not, has heard of the Israelites wandering for forty years in the wilderness. They had been in slavery in Egypt and had been crying out to God for deliverance. God heard their prayer and called Moses to go as His Ambassador to lead them out of bondage. He took them to a land of blessing that flowed with milk and honey. Aren't God's illustrations interesting? How often He uses food in the scriptures to make a point. After all of the years crying for deliverance, at the first sign of difficulty, the Israelites began murmuring and complaining. They asked to go back to Egypt. At the Red Sea, they told Moses it was entirely his fault that they had gotten into this situation. They asked, "Why didn't you leave us alone serving the Egyptians?" The mentality of being a slave was easier than walking by faith. They had been taken out of Egypt, but Egypt was still very much in them.

It is interesting that God called them into Egypt originally because of their lack of food. Now, that was all they could think about. They would rather go back to where they had been slaves. That was easier than making responsible choices to be obedient to what God was doing to deliver them. Upon arriving at the very border of the Promised Land the first time, they drew back, because of fear and doubt. They would not believe the evidence before their very eyes that the land was good. They could not believe that God would make them able! It had only taken God one day to bring them out of Egypt, but it took the next forty years to get Egypt out of them.

God is calling all of us out of being bound to a life of overeating. He is calling us into a promised land of freedom. It is not a land of lack, but a place of balance where everything works together for our good. Until we are able to have the slave mentality worked out of us, we resist having to make responsible choices. That is why the discipline of the wilderness seems so hard. But, it was never God's intention to leave us there. He only intends for us to be in the wilderness long enough to have Egypt worked out of our lives. We know that the discipline of the wilderness is coming to an end when we don't even notice that we are being disciplined anymore. Then and only then are we ready to enter this new land of freedom. As we enter in, the ability to make responsible choices becomes a part of our new nature. Again, God will honor His word and bring us through.

Prayer

Heavenly Father, I thank you that you are taking me out of bondage and into freedom. Forgive me for murmuring and complaining. I refuse to despise the discipline of the wilderness. Today, I surrender myself completely. I know you are making me able to walk in a new lifestyle of responsible choices. I will lose weight as an outward sign of my being set free. I declare by faith that I will never go back, in Jesus' name, amen.

—Day 31—
Selling Your Birthright for a Bowl of Soup

Daily Opening Prayer

Heavenly Father, I come to you in the name of my Lord and Savior Jesus Christ to present myself as a living sacrifice, which is my reasonable service. Cleanse me today from the sin of willfulness and fill me with your holiness. Today, I choose to burn the fat on the fire. Accept this offering and enable me to live a self-controlled life by the power of the Holy Spirit who lives in me. I refuse to despise and resist the disciplining of the Lord, which demonstrates His great love for me. I ask this in Jesus' name, amen.

Almost everyone has heard the story of Jacob and Esau. Each man was wrong in how he did things, but Esau's problem went deeper. "Make sure that no one is immoral or godless like Esau. He traded his birthright as the oldest son for a single meal." (Hebrew 12: 16) New Living Translation. The King James Version states that he was a fornicator and a profane man. Here the word fornicator means someone who sells himself or herself. The word profane in this context means someone who has contempt. We see Esau as a person who only wanted to serve his own needs. He wanted those needs met instantly. He had no vision for the things of God. If something required discipline from him, he ignored it. His choice cost him his birthright.

Our priorities are backwards, too. When we choose immediate gratification, the consequences of our actions sell us into bondage. We will never be able to eat enough to satisfy the cravings in our souls with temporal food. If we feed our inner man first, both our souls and our bodies will be satisfied. "For he that soweth to his flesh shall of the flesh reap corruption; but, he that soweth to the Spirit shall of the Spirit reap life everlasting." (Galatians 6:8) King James Version Again, God works from the inside out.

We are overweight because it has felt better to eat what we wanted, when we wanted it, rather than practice any kind of discipline. We have stayed stuffed and satisfied on things that perish rather than feeding ourselves on things that have lasting benefit. In John 6:27 Jesus tells us our efforts should not be toward the food that perishes, but toward the food that brings eternal life. When we are born again into God's family we immediately inherit Jesus' own birthright. This covers every area of our lives. The Bible tells us that God has given us everything that pertains to life and godliness. Isn't it sad that we spend so much time being shortsighted in choosing things that don't last instead of choosing what will give us lasting benefit? We have chosen pleasure in the things that immediately satisfy rather than the discipline needed to change us permanently. By doing this we feed and strengthen the habits in our old nature. This makes us fat. As the satisfaction of the quick fix wears off we quickly want to eat again. It is a cycle of death.

The Bible says there is a hunger that leads to life and there is a hunger that leads to death. God means to always give us our daily bread. If we keep choosing to overindulge in food that only temporarily satisfies us, we cheat ourselves out of the eternal satisfaction that is ours as a birthright. Let's stop selling our birthright, folks. We are shortchanging ourselves and living a life devoid of God's best blessings. Let's begin to value our birthright and take full advantage of what Jesus purchased for us. Let's stop making the temporal meal our priority when the true priority is eating the Bread of Life. As we do this God will begin to change the inside of us, which will cause outward weight loss through the fruit in our lives of temperance and self-control. We will have our real hunger satisfied first by this eternal Bread of Life.

Prayer

Heavenly Father, I confess to you that I have tried to fill up the hunger of my soul with earthly food. I realize my real need is to feast on Jesus as the Bread of Life. Forgive me for making wrong choices and help me get my priorities straight. As I do this, you will strengthen my inner man. I know that when I am full inside, I will not continue to desire to overeat. Thank you for setting me free. My old appetites will no longer have power over me. I praise you for this deliverance. I ask this in Jesus' name, amen.

—Day 32—
Let Patience Have Its Perfect Work

Daily Opening Prayer
Heavenly Father, I come to you in the name of my Lord and Savior Jesus Christ to present myself as a living sacrifice, which is my reasonable service. Cleanse me today from the sin of willfulness and fill me with your holiness. Today, I choose to burn the fat on the fire. Accept this offering and enable me to live a self-controlled life by the power of the Holy Spirit who lives in me. I refuse to despise and resist the disciplining of the Lord, which demonstrates His great love for me. I ask this in Jesus' name, amen.

In today's world the desire for instant answers has turned the word **patience** into a four-letter word. The Lord calls the word patience a virtue. Virtue means a positive value that shows in your life. In James 1 we are told to be joyful when different kinds of trouble come our way. We are told that this makes our patience grow. In this text patience and endurance are interchangeable. James promises that when we have allowed our endurance to grow we will be strong in character and ready for anything.

Dr. David Goodwin, founder of Christian Life Worship Center in Des Moines, Iowa, teaches that patience is a weapon against the enemy. Patience allows us enough time for the enemy's deception to be revealed. How many times in our "fight against fat" do we think, I'm not getting anywhere? Why bother? I'm going to be fat for the rest of my life so I'm just not going to care. Then we go find the nearest fast food fix and stuff ourselves until the ache goes away. We say it and then we go out and make it happen. It's a vicious circle and causes us to remain locked into our miserable, overweight existence.

When we begin to exercise patience, it's like starting a physical exercise program. At first our muscles hurt, because they haven't been used. As we exercise patience, it hurts, too. We must remember there is always going to be resistance from our flesh as well as from the enemy. Patience is the very thing that lets us follow through until we see the answer. In Hebrews 10: 35-36 we read, "Do not throw away this confident trust in the Lord, no matter what happens. Remember the great reward it brings you. Patient endurance is what you need now, so you will continue to do God's will. Then you will receive all that He has promised." (New Living Translation)

Our confidence is in the Lord. If we look at ourselves or at our circumstances we will become easily defeated. It makes us susceptible to the enemy's lies. Later in Hebrews chapter 12 we are told to run with patience the race that is set before us looking unto Jesus as the author and finisher of our faith. We fail and circumstances disappoint us, but Jesus never fails. When we focus on Him, He gives us the ability to forget about time and let patience have its perfect work. We are not disappointed when we look to Him. Let us continue on exercising this great weapon of patience to the end.

Prayer

Heavenly Father, thank you for providing me with the power I need to exercise Patience. This comes through the indwelling presence of the Holy Spirit. Forgive me when I allow anything to break my focus and stop me from following you to the end of the course set before me. Today, I will pick up this weapon, remembering that my confidence is in you. As I do this, I will receive your promise. I will see my life bear the fruit of patient endurance. This will change my inner man and as a result I will lose weight. Thank you for this victory, in Jesus' name, amen.

—Day 33—

Be Moldable Clay—God Will Reshape You

Daily Opening Prayer

Heavenly Father, I come to you in the name of my Lord and Savior Jesus Christ to present myself as a living sacrifice, which is my reasonable service. Cleanse me today from the sin of willfulness and fill me with your holiness. Today, I choose to burn the fat on the fire. Accept this offering and enable me to live a self-controlled life by the power of the Holy Spirit who lives in me. I refuse to despise and resist the disciplining of the Lord, which demonstrates His great love for me. I ask this in Jesus' name, amen.

Have you ever thought, *I hate my shape—I wish I didn't look like this*? God is ready and willing to reshape you. As with everything God does, this must start inside you first. In Jeremiah 18 we read how the prophet was told by the Lord to go to the potter's house and watch how he made his pots. As Jeremiah watched he saw the potter squash a marred pot he was working on and begin to reshape it. This is a picture of how the Lord works with us. At times we can feel as though our lives are being totally squashed. This is not to destroy us, but to reshape us. Have you ever worked with clay? First, you must carefully center it on the wheel. Then, the clay must be repeatedly slammed down hard to get the air pockets out. The potter begins to spin the wheel placing one hand inside the pot while the other hand presses from the outside. This is how he hollows out the center. During the whole process he is adding water to keep the clay pliable.

We are like the clay and God is the potter. We have to be confronted with some harsh realities before we become willing to let Him shape us into a vessel He can use. This can be compared to the way the potter slams the clay. Next, He carefully centers us in Jesus, just as the clay was centered on the wheel. The spinning can be likened to our constant repentance as the water of the word is applied to our lives. The press of His fingers is the Holy Spirit using the word to mold us. He presses from the inside to form our shape, while He presses from the outside to smooth away the rough edges. With God, the shaping of the inside is just as important as the shaping of the outside!

We must see the reason for the vessel of our lives to be properly shaped. In 2 Corinthians 4 the apostle Paul tells us that we have the treasure of the glory of God, Jesus Christ, in our earthen vessels. This is so everyone can see that the power rests with God and not in us. If we let God shape our vessel, not only will we contain His glory, He will then shape our outside into something we are pleased with. Then we will be ready for His use.

Prayer

Heavenly Father, I thank you that you never throw the clay away. You already see the finished vessel. Forgive me for trying to tell you how to form me and resisting your loving pressure. Today, I will yield myself wholly to you for you to shape and mold me for your pleasure. Your word tells me you know the plan you have for me to give me a hope and a future. I praise you that as I release myself into your hands you will change me both inside and out. I ask this in Jesus' name, amen.

—Day 34—
Embrace Correction

Daily Opening Prayer

Heavenly Father, I come to you in the name of my Lord and Savior Jesus Christ to present myself as a living sacrifice, which is my reasonable service. Cleanse me today from the sin of willfulness and fill me with your holiness. Today, I choose to burn the fat on the fire. Accept this offering and enable me to live a self-controlled life by the power of the Holy Spirit who lives in me. I refuse to despise and resist the disciplining of the Lord, which demonstrates His great love for me. I ask this in Jesus' name, amen.

How much do you hate to be corrected? When someone tells you you're doing something the wrong way, does it make you angry? Are you able to be objective and consider what you are being told or do you immediately reject it?

When the Israelites wandered in the wilderness, God was doing all He could to correct them. He wanted them to be prepared to enter the Promised Land. He knew their hearts were not right. In His wonderful wisdom He knew He could instantly change their outward circumstances, but that would never have lasted. God wanted eternal change inside of His people. He used correction as the tool for change. Because they rebelled, they all died in the wilderness. They thought the bondage in which they had been living in Egypt was better than receiving the correction from the Lord that would set them free.

When we are living our own way, choosing to do our own thing and correction comes, we get mad. We have chosen to indulge our flesh to a point that our flesh is in control. It demands to be constantly fed and rejects all efforts to stop it. As a result, our bodies become overweight and we become slaves to our appetites. We lose our health, our mobility, and our self-respect.

Let's use the example of someone flying an airplane. When the plane is on target and begins to drift out of alignment, because of wind pressure and atmospheric conditions, the pilot corrects the plane. He does this to ensure that the plane stays on course and safely reaches its destination.

In our lives God has given us the Holy Spirit as our Counselor and Guide. He gives us correction and instruction so we can stay on course. In the midst of changing circumstances, He uses each day's situations to keep us focused in the right direction. We must choose to allow Him to do this. It is the enemy and our flesh that cause us to think we are being condemned when we are actually being corrected. God's Word tells us in Romans 8 that there is no condemnation to them who are in Christ Jesus; who walk not after the flesh.

It doesn't matter how many times we are corrected, it only matters that we embrace each correction. We are all at different places in our walk with God. He meets each of us right where we are. In Proverbs 15:32 we are told that when we reject correction we harm ourselves, but when we listen to correction we begin to understand. Let's begin to embrace correction today and see outward weight loss as a direct result.

Prayer

Heavenly Father, I thank you that you gave me the Holy Spirit to be with me and in me. He guides me with gentle correction as I yield to him. Forgive me when I become proud and stiff-necked, refusing to yield. Today, I fully and freely submit myself to you that I might receive your correction. Instruct me that I might live. I praise you that in Jesus there is no condemnation. I have liberty to walk in newness of life. Thank You that as I let you make these changes in my heart I will see my body change as well. Thank you for your wonderful faithfulness. I ask this in Jesus' name, amen.

—Day 35—
And the Word Became Flesh
(or the Lack Of)

Daily Opening Prayer

Heavenly Father, I come to you in the name of my Lord and Savior Jesus Christ to present myself as a living sacrifice, which is my reasonable service. Cleanse me today from the sin of willfulness and fill me with your holiness. Today, I choose to burn the fat on the fire. Accept this offering and enable me to live a self-controlled life by the power of the Holy Spirit who lives in me. I refuse to despise and resist the disciplining of the Lord, which demonstrates His great love for me. I ask this in Jesus' name, amen.

Let us consider creation. God thought of what He wanted to create and spoke it out. As a result the real physical world came into existence. He created man in a natural physical body. Because we are natural, we have a tendency to want to work from the outside in. God's purpose in everything He does is to go from the spiritual into the natural.

God always plans to change the outward appearance; He just does it His way. God is always available to us in this natural Kingdom. Because we can't see Him right now, we are afraid He doesn't care about the outward appearance of things. That's just not true! God simply works backwards to the world system.

God produces change in the outward appearance because He cares about what's important to us. He starts on the inside first, because he wants a lasting change. God only asks that we begin to prepare the inside of us to fit the new bodies He is preparing for us in His Kingdom. As we are changed inside, our outward appearance begins to conform here in this world to the image of Jesus himself. We lose outward fat and gain it inside in our spiritual man.

God truly wants us to see ourselves the way He does. Through His constant love we can relax and know that He who has begun a good work within us will perform it until the day of Jesus Christ (Philippians 1:6). "...let us lay aside every weight, and the sin that doth so easily beset us, and let us run with patience the race that be set before us, looking unto Jesus the author and finisher of our faith..." (Hebrews 12:1-2) King James Version Remember always that God finishes everything he starts!

Prayer

Heavenly Father, I thank you that I can rely on you to help me complete what I start. Forgive me for thinking you don't care about what matters so much to me. I see from your word you have answered my prayer and are at work within me to change my inner man. This will cause my outward man to show it. Thank You for permanent change in both places. I praise you that when you are finished, my outward appearance will be pleasing to us both. I ask this in Jesus' name, amen.

—Day 36—
Stop Believing a Lie

Daily Opening Prayer

Heavenly Father, I come to you in the name of my Lord and Savior Jesus Christ to present myself as a living sacrifice, which is my reasonable service. Cleanse me today from the sin of willfulness and fill me with your holiness. Today, I choose to burn the fat on the fire. Accept this offering and enable me to live a self-controlled life by the power of the Holy Spirit who lives in me. I refuse to despise and resist the disciplining of them Lord, which demonstrates His great love for me. I ask this in Jesus' name, amen.

The amount of freedom we have from bondage in our lives is directly proportionate to the amount of obedience we have to God's truth. The amount of bondage we have in our lives is directly related to the amount of lies we still believe.

In John 8:44 Jesus exposes Satan as the Father of lies. He was a murderer from the beginning and has always hated the truth. Earlier in John 8:31, Jesus taught that if we are truly His disciples we will continue to obey His teachings. We will then know the truth and the truth will set us free. "For the Scriptures say,"If you want a happy life and good days, keep your tongue from speaking evil, and keep your lips from telling lies.'' (1 Peter 3: 10) New Living Translation. These principles are there to help us succeed.

Our entire walk as a Christian is meant to train us to recognize the difference between God's truth and the enemy's lies. The Prince of the power of the air, Satan, controls the world in which we live. In 2 Corinthians 4:4 we are told that Satan, as the god of this world, is blinding men's minds and causing them to believe a lie. God counsels us to not be conformed to this world, but we are to be transformed by the renewing of our minds (Romans 12:2).

As always, God works from the inside out. Whatever we believe in our hearts is what we will do in our lives. If we believe we cannot succeed at losing weight, we believe a lie. If our hearts haven't been changed, we will continue to follow diets, programs, and medical advice aimed at changing only our outward appearance. Inwardly, we are programmed to expect failure. You say to yourself, *I'll try, but it won't work—it's never worked before.* This lie is from the enemy of your soul who wants to kill, steal, and destroy your life. He has deceived you.

In direct opposition to the lies of the enemy, we have God's truth. In Philippians 4:13 God, reveals His truth to us. He tells us we can do all things with the help of Christ who gives us the inward strength to do it. This includes losing weight! Every time the lie is rerun in our minds we have to make the conscious choice to believe God instead. We choose to believe the truth, reject the lie, and continue doing His word. This is how the truth sets us free.

Prayer

Heavenly Father, I thank you, Lord, that you have made your truth available to me through your living word, Jesus Christ. He is the Life that exposes every lie. He is the Truth that tells me what to do, and He is the Way that shows me how to do it. Forgive me that I have chosen to believe a lie because it was easier than being responsible. As I present myself to you as a living sacrifice your word will transform my mind. You make me able to obey. Today, I choose to walk in your truth. I praise you that as I continue to walk in your truth, your truth will continually set me free. I will lose weight as the outward show of my inward obedience. I ask this in Jesus' name, amen.

—Day 37—
Thou Shalt Have No Other Gods Before Me

Daily Opening Prayer

Heavenly Father, I come to you in the name of my Lord and Savior Jesus Christ to present myself as a living sacrifice, which is my reasonable service. Cleanse me today from the sin of willfulness and fill me with your holiness. Today, I choose to burn the fat on the fire. Accept this offering and enable me to live a self-controlled life by the power of the Holy Spirit who lives in me. I refuse to despise and resist the disciplining of the Lord, which demonstrates His great love for me. I ask this in Jesus' name, amen.

God created man to be the ruler of this world. In the Garden of Eden, Adam and Eve chose to eat what they had been told not to. This brought sin upon all mankind and gave the rulership over to Satan. The Bible says that Satan is now the god of this world. Man sold himself into bondage by choosing to believe Satan's lies. Actually, they chose to make their appetite their god by yielding to Satan's suggestion.

Jesus came and lived a totally submitted life. He became the perfect sacrifice and broke the power of sin over us. Now, through salvation and the indwelling presence of the Holy Spirit, we have become God's children again. Now we can choose to follow His ways. Each time we choose to follow our appetites instead of God's instruction, we make that appetite god over us. The longer we serve that god, the stronger its control becomes.

Romans 6:16 reminds us that to whatever we yield ourselves, we become its servants. Before we are born again, we can only hear from our flesh, our bodily appetites. Through acceptance of Jesus Christ, our spiritual man is made alive and able to hear from God. The conflict occurs in our minds because we have to choose which information we are going to follow. We must decide, do we want to be ruled by our appetites and continually reap destruction, or do we want to choose God and His truth and live? (Read Philippians 3:18-21).

When we follow God's way, He begins recreating our bodies now. We don't have to wait until we get to Heaven. We can choose now not to have any other god, but the one who loves us, gave Himself for us, and wants to bless us with bodies that help us serve Him.

Prayer

Heavenly Father, I thank you that you have given back to me the ability to hear and understand your truth. Forgive me for continuing to follow the desires of my flesh rather than choosing to obey your instructions. Today, I will submit myself to you as a living sacrifice. I declare I will serve you and have no other gods before you. Each time I feel the compulsion to overeat I will submit myself to you, resist the temptation, and watch my body change. Thank you, that as I continue to choose your ways, you will change me inside. I will see my body lose weight as the outward sign of my inner obedience. We praise you for your wonderful love, mercy, and grace and in Jesus' name I ask this, amen.

—Day 38—
Be Addicted to Jesus

Daily Opening Prayer

Heavenly Father, I come to you in the name of my Lord and Savior Jesus Christ to present myself as a living sacrifice, which is my reasonable service. Cleanse me today from the sin of willfulness and fill me with your holiness. Today, I choose to burn the fat on the fire. Accept this offering and enable me to live a self-controlled life to the power of the Holy Spirit who lives in me. I refuse to despise and resist the disciplining of the Lord, which demonstrates His great love for me. I ask this in Jesus' name, amen.

In today's world the word addiction has become so familiar that even our little children know what it means. Insurance companies recognize it as a disease. In the true sense, addiction really is a DIS—EASE. Man was never created to be at the mercy of creation. Man was created to be at the mercy of God. He was created to crave and be ruled over by God alone. The Rev. Andre Brooks called this a "dominion flip." In Genesis we are told that man was given dominion over all of God's creation; birds, plants, and animals. After the fall into sin, Satan now uses these very things to take dominion over man.

We are all aware of drug addiction, alcohol addiction, and sexual addiction. Today, we are going to consider food addiction. Have you ever had that bag of cookies, candy, or containers of ice cream call your name? Have you ever eaten to fullness, but had to have just one more helping, because it tasted so good? Where do all these food items come from? They come from creation. Man is basically a spiritual being living in a physical body. He was created in God's image to crave fellowship with his Creator. When sin entered in, creation began ruling man through the appetites of his body. This always causes bondages.

Jesus Christ lived, died, and rose again to reverse this flip and give us back the dominion we lost. Through submission to Jesus, God alone can once again rule us. When we continue to live with harmful addictions, we are influenced mostly by our flesh and its cravings for the things of this world. When our appetites rule we are never satisfied.

God craved fellowship so He created us. Because we are created in His image, we also have a craving as part of our makeup. Satan has used this to deceive us. He has caused us to crave the creation rather than the Creator. Since Jesus took back the dominion at Calvary, we again have authority to rule over creation in His Name. We need to start with our own appetites. Let's become addicted to God and live a victorious life, set free to enjoy God's creation as He intended.

Prayer
Heavenly Father, I thank you that I can choose my addiction today. Forgive me for choosing to give in to my fleshly appetites. I repent for allowing my flesh to rule my life. Today, I submit myself to you as a living sacrifice. I ask you to renew in me the craving for You I was created to have. Thank you that as I am satisfied by you in my inner man, I will be set free from the desire for any other addiction. These choices will produce eternal change inside and out. I ask this in Jesus' name, amen.

—Day 39—
Beware the Root of Bitterness

Daily Opening Prayer

Heavenly Father, I come to you in the name of my Lord and Savior Jesus Christ to present myself as a living sacrifice, which is my reasonable service. Cleanse me today from the sin of willfulness and fill me with your holiness. Today, I choose to burn the fat on the fire. Accept this offering and enable me to live a self-controlled life by the power of the Holy Spirit who lives in me. I refuse to despise and resist the disciplining of the Lord, which demonstrates His great love for me. I ask this in Jesus' name, amen.

Have you ever been bitter because of your appearance? Haven't we all looked at someone and said, "Why can't I look like her or him?" Let's consider the possible correlation between these bitter, resentful feelings and the choices we make in our everyday lives.

Let's take a mental journey to one of our social gatherings. How many times do we find ourselves fellowshipping around a table piled with high-caloric foods, empty of nutritional value? Invariably someone will hold their hand out over the food (after the blessing) and curse the calories. We all laugh and feel safe now to be gluttons and eat until we're stuffed. The minute someone mentions that this is possibly excessive, we become self-righteously indignant. The usual reply is, "After all, we are fellowshipping in the Lord!"

What happens is, the more we sit and eat, the more we have to sit on! What we asked God to bless has become a curse. Let's look at God's Word. "Look after each other so that none of you will miss out on the special favor of God. Watch out that no bitter root of unbelief rises up among you, for whenever it springs up; many are corrupted by its poison." (Hebrews 12; 15) New Living Translation It seems that the person cautioning against excess was actually following the scripture. We must remember that the mighty God we serve teaches temperance and self-control as a lifestyle.

In Deuteronomy the Bible talks about the root of bitterness. Moses reminded the Israelites of their covenant relationship with God. If they chose to follow His ways, they were promised that blessings would follow them. If they chose their own way, curses would beset them.

In Deuteronomy 29:18 Moses warned against doing your own thing and expecting God to bless it. Isn't this what we are doing every time we curse the calories and continue to gorge ourselves? We think, because we've gathered in His name, we can indulge our flesh and be protected from the consequences. This works great until we look in a mirror. The lie is revealed in all of its ugliness. We must stop feeding ourselves with sugarcoated garbage, both in our souls and in our bodies. Let's not be like Esau who exchanged his birthright for food. God has something better in mind for his children.

Prayer

Heavenly Father, I thank you for how your word reveals the truth. Forgive me for rejecting your way and thinking you should bless my rebellion. I realize your blessing is only available to me as I obey your word. Today, I repent for making your word of no effect. Help me to exercise the discipline and self-control that will cause any root of bitterness to die. I thank you and praise you that your help will always lead me to life and health. As I make wise choices, I will be changed inside and lose weight as an outward sign of my obedience. I ask this in Jesus' name, amen.

—Day 40—
Without a Vision, People Perish

Daily Opening Prayer

Heavenly Father, I come to you in the name of my Lord and Savior Jesus Christ to present myself as a living sacrifice, which is my reasonable service. Cleanse me today from the sin of willfulness and fill me with your holiness. Today, I choose to burn the fat on the fire. Accept this offering and enable me to live a self-controlled life by the power of the Holy Spirit who lives in me. I refuse to despise and resist the disciplining of the Lord, which demonstrates His great love for me. I ask this in Jesus' name, amen.

Years ago, I found myself driving through the foothills surrounding Las Vegas, Nevada. It was very dark. There were no stars to break the night sky. It was an area where there were no houses or farms; just complete stillness. It gave me the eerie sense of being caught up in the middle of nothingness with nowhere to go.

Suddenly, I came up over the last hill and the whole "Valley of Lights", that is, Las Vegas, appeared. It provided an instant vision of life and dispelled the cold feeling of being alone and helpless. I don't think I'll ever forget the intense feeling of relief that ran through me.

Often in the midst of our everyday lives we experience this same sense of nothingness, or going nowhere. As we look around there doesn't seem to be anything to focus on. We can't seem to find a direction or a purpose. When this happens we feel helpless, hopeless, and depressed. We become lethargic and almost unable to function. When we try to look down the road, it seems so far to our goal that we don't even want to begin the journey.

When I was driving in that Nevada darkness, I couldn't see my long-range goal. In order to get to my destination safely I had to keep my eyes on the immediate, short-term goals that I knew would lead me to my desired end. I watched for road signs, mile markers, warning signs, and the possibility of nocturnal critters running into my path.

On our weight loss journey, when we try to look too far ahead, we get frightened and inpatient. We just can't seem to get a vision of our bodies changed into that slimmer, healthier form we desire to have. Let's remember, the journey can be started more than once. If something happens to interrupt our journey, we don't have to go back to the beginning; we just go on from where we are. In fact, in long journeys, people sometimes take a break just to rest. We can do some sightseeing or just appreciate how far we've come. The key is to keep the vision of where you want to go while you're paying attention to what's right in front of you at the moment. This provides the balance necessary for a smooth trip.

God's Word tells us that without a vision, people perish. The whole meaning of vision here includes some built-in restraints. "When people do not accept divine guidance, they run wild. But whoever obeys the law is happy." (Proverbs 29: 18) New Living translation God has provided wisdom and instruction through his word as our road signs. It warns us of possible places for accidents, detours, and delays. It tells us how to avoid these hindrances so we can reach our destination with a minimal amount of problems. The road signs keep you informed of how much further you need to go and if you are still headed in the right direction. When we view our journey through Jesus Christ, we don't have to worry about getting to our final destination. We can rest in following His instructions. We can be assured because His love for us will keep our vision unclouded, and we will not perish.

Prayer

Heavenly Father, thank you for providing me with both a vision of where to go and how to get there. Forgive me when I refuse to be guided by your word and as a result become lost or stalled. Help me to remember that in Jesus Christ I can begin again right where I am. Today, I will pay attention and yield to your instructions. I praise you that you will keep me on the right path, and I will reach my goal destination. I will lose weight and keep it off. I ask this in Jesus' name, amen.

THANK YOU FROM OUR HEARTS

We want to thank everyone who so graciously agreed to read, critique, comments on and pray. Many times it is these wonderful people who make things go smoothly, keep the enemy at bay and allow connected thought! It would be difficult to name them all, but you know who you are.

Lynn Montgomery currently resides with her husband of twenty-seven years, Paul, in central Florida. Lynn is co-founder and former director of Life Limited to Faith in Jesus Christ, a faith-based community outreach center in Des Moines, Iowa. In her capacity as a leader with Life Limited, Inc., she provided counseling, food, clothing, shelter, and emergency funds on a regular basis. She worked in conjunction with the Fifth Judicial District's Community Service Sentencing Program assisting ex-offenders back into society.

While working at KWKY Christian Radio, Lynn hosted her own interview show. Her program, "The Bond of Unity Hour," played host to many recognized celebrities from the Christian community. Lynn attended Open Bible College and holds a certificate in the "Competent to Counsel Program". She has become a popular speaker for women's groups throughout the Central Iowa area.

Margaret Thomas is a former adviser to board members and part of the counseling staff for Life Limited to Faith in Jesus Christ. She worked tirelessly as the Christian Education Director for Christian Life Worship Center, Des Moines, Iowa. Today, Margaret stays busy caring for her family and works in her position as Christian Ed Director for the Faith Family Church.